THE HAPPINESS WORKOUT

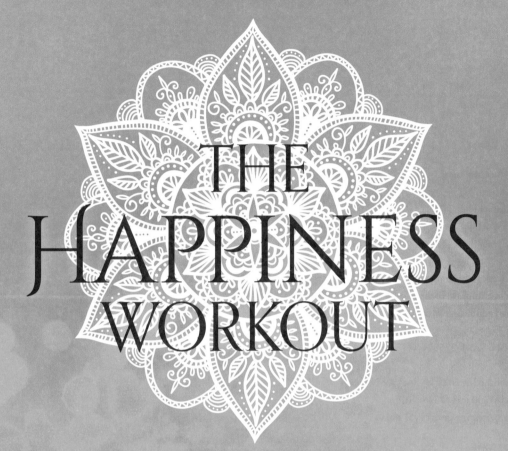

THE HAPPINESS WORKOUT

Learn how to optimise confidence,
creativity and your brain!

NOA BELLING

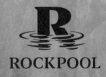

ROCKPOOL

INTRODUCTION

*'The more you invest in happiness, the
more happiness will invest in you.'*
ALAN COHEN

It is common knowledge that regular exercise helps to keep your body strong, flexible and healthy. What might not be known is that the same applies to happiness that can also be strengthened and toned by practising particular kinds of exercises. How is this so? The answer lies in your ability to manufacture happiness from the inside out by influencing the bio-chemistry associated with happiness. What kinds of exercises strengthen and tone it? This is what the book is all about.

Understanding the bio-chemistry of happiness involves understanding that happiness can be experienced in different ways. It can be a sense of peace and deeper meaning. It can be love and harmony. It can be courage and a strong sense of purpose. It can be excitement and passion. Each have their own bio-chemical signature and all dance together in a life well lived.

The bio-chemicals representing these different qualities of happiness include serotonin, testosterone, dopamine and oxytocin. This book hones in on specific physical skills that can stimulate this bio-chemistry, namely grounding, strength, fluidity, agility, flexibility and warmheartedness. These physical skills not only can influence happiness, they can also stimulate associated qualities such as resilience, compassion, confidence and creativity. They can also literally tone your nervous system to promote and sustain happiness with an added bonus of optimising brain functioning too.

This does not undermine your stresses and challenging feelings such as sadness, anger, shame and fear. What it does is support your ability to navigate life's ups and downs with greater skill. For example, the skills of this book can help you connect with greater peacefulness, acceptance, courage, proactive energy and motivation, resilience and compassion to help you through trying times. You are also able to directly influence the bio-chemistry of stress, such as adrenaline and cortisol, as the main bio-chemical culprits that can cloud your happiness. To keep your stress bio-chemistry at bay targeted physical strategies are offered to help you bounce back into a more confident and creative flow.

The kind of exercise required to strengthen and tone happiness is exercise with a difference. To start with there is a variety of short physical techniques that take just a few seconds or a couple of minutes to apply, and are intended for inserting now and again in your usual day. They are referred to as short practices or quick tips and are interspersed through the different sections of the book. These are invitations to align with and reinforce happiness in small, accessible daily ways. This could be as simple as pausing now and again to shift posture, release tension, refocus attention or deepen breathing in ways that are proven to stimulate feel-good bio-chemistry. Many of these interventions can be used anytime and anywhere, even at work or while on the go and results can be quick. In a matter of minutes, or sometimes seconds, it is possible to feel noticeably stronger, more positive and happier. This formula of small amounts of time invested regularly is backed by neuroscience as an effective way to create lasting change in brain and body.

The short practices can be enhanced when you use the longer happiness workouts also on offer. The workouts are designed to promote physical fitness while specifically building the physical skills of happiness. The workouts are not essential if you do not feel physically up for them although if your physical ability allows, they can significantly boost your relationship with the physical skills. Workouts are about 20 minutes each, can be practised in the comfort of your home and are adaptable to different fitness levels and physical abilities. Used for physical fitness, they are recommended for use 3-5 days per week, allowing for rest days in between and with the possibility to use any workout that you like repeatedly or alternately. If you have an existing exercise practice, you can use relevant workouts when you feel the need to boost the particular physical skill. In this you can either replace or supplement your usual exercise program. This will depend on your preference and your exercise advice from a health professional when applicable.

The most important recommendation is to practise something regularly, or to practise regularly when the need arises. This could involve applying a short practice or quick tip now and again through the day or investing in the longer workouts or both. Accumulatively this can anchor your life in a happiness that is deeply rooted in your body, with feel-good chemicals produced in greater abundance and a smile more readily on your face. Over time this can rewire your brain with new neural pathways so that happiness becomes a default setting. This happiness feels calm and peaceful at times, exciting and motivating at other times, while helping to steer your life in uplifting, heartfelt and meaningful directions.

Then when you might go through trying times and happiness feels far away, which can be a natural part of life's ebb and flow, you might be quicker to remember your physical abilities for stimulating supportive bio-chemistry. With this you can grow more skilful at bouncing back into the inner peace, resilience, courage and compassion that are always available to you.

With a uniquely body-based approach, you might ask why working through the body is so effective? The answer lies in the way that your body can bypass thoughts and emotions and trick your brain into believing that you are stronger and happier. To get a sense of this, try this out. Slouch you posture and notice how it makes you feel and what kinds of thoughts come to mind. Maintaining this posture, try to feel happy. How did that go? Now right your posture, take a nice deep breath into your chest and hold your head up high. How does this make you feel and what kind of thoughts spring to mind? Maintaining this posture, try to feel sad. How did that go? Probably not so well because of the way your feelings tend to follow your body. Finally add a small smile to your face and invite your whole body to smile along with you and notice how this might shift your mind and mood. This book is full of these kinds of tricks that leverage your body to hack your brain, shift how you feel and influence how you respond to daily situations. Effects can be immediate while over time also building enduring habits of happiness.

The stories that weave through the book are true stories of how people have worked with and integrated the physical skills of happiness into their lives. These stories have been adapted from my private psychotherapy and corporate consulting practices and sometimes they are conglomerate examples weaving together similar stories of a few people. I am grateful to each person whose story has contributed to the material of this book. All names and some details have been changed to protect their identities.

Section and Chapter Overview

The first section introduces the bio-chemistry of happiness. Chapter 1 hones in on the various bio-chemicals involved in happiness as well as those stimulated when we feel stressed. Chapter 2 explores how this bio-chemistry, with its different experiential qualities, works together to maintain a 'happy balance'. In this chapter there are opportunities to assess yourself in relation to which qualities are strong in you at this time and which might benefit from being developed. This can guide you to the chapters and physical skills that you most need or wish to focus on at the time. Chapter 3 introduces the physical skills of happiness and offers another opportunity for self-assessment in relation to these skills to further clarify which are strong and which could benefit from development.

The following chapters 4–11 dive into each of the physical skills and how they support happiness in distinct ways. These sections are filled with short practices and quick tips for shorter and longer term gain. Also included is supportive information and some of the science that underpins these skills. Relevant workout recommendations are flagged at the end of the chapters. The aim is to build understanding and physical skill in simple ways that are accessible to all ages and levels of fitness. Chapters 4–5 focus on the physical skill of grounding associated with serotonin. Chapters 6–7 hone in on strength associated with testosterone. Chapters 8–9 focus on fluidity, agility and flexibility associated with dopamine. Chapters 10–11 are dedicated to warmheartedness associated with oxytocin.

Following this are chapters 12–13 exploring ways to bounce back from stress and maintain happiness in physical ways that promote your feel-good bio-chemistry. Chapter 12 offers resources for leveraging the body to bounce back from stress as well as placing this in the context of your nervous system and what it means to tone your nervous system for happiness. In so doing you can gain a better understanding of your stress responses and what it takes to keep stress hormones such as cortisol and adrenaline at bay. Chapter 13 explores the enlivening combination of grounding and fluidity as the basis for posture that is conducive to both health and happiness. Included are simple physical practices that can be used at home, work or while out and about, with options to release tension and free up posture while sitting and standing.

The book concludes with two appendices. Appendix 1 is a quick reference guide to all the physical practices contained throughout the book. It contains a menu of all the short practices, quick tips and longer workouts for you to peruse and choose from according to what you need or would like to develop at different times. Also included is a guide to common emotions and feelings, such as anxiety, worry, depression, emptiness, shame, low self-esteem, chronic anger, irritability, melancholy and fear, that tend to go with different stress responses to guide you to supportive practices.

With the menu of Appendix 1 you can also design your own workout plan and choose from the exercises that interest you or that you feel you need at the time. You might also come to identify a toolkit that can work well in different circumstances, such as when you are at home with family or at work and preparing to go into an important meeting or presentation, or when you need a boost to your creative thinking. This appendix also contains a set of challenges, including 3 day, 7 day and 21 day challenges to motivate your use of the various happiness-boosting skills.

Appendix 2 contains a photographic, step-by-step guide to all the workouts for developing the physical skills of happiness. This includes some posture adaptations and options for different physical abilities.

To Best Use This Book

It is recommended that you first read through each of the chapters, or at least the chapters that you feel you could benefit from most at this time, perhaps based on your self-assessments in the opening chapters. As you read through it is recommended that you try out the various exercises. This will help you to understand the exercises in the context of supporting information and experiment with their effect. Over time it is recommended that you carve out time to read through and familiarise yourself with all of the physical skills on offer in this book that can support your holistic happiness. This will familiarise you with the practices on offer in the Appendix 1 menu designed to keep your happiness flowing and fresh.

The hope is also that you dip into this book over and over again and use the exercises for many years to come as empowering and uplifting support through life's ups and downs.

It is useful to add that the brain tends to thrive on a good balance between familiarity and novelty. For familiarity, it is important to focus on particular techniques for a period of time to reap maximum rewards. For this, you are welcome to use your favourite exercises over and over again until they start to come naturally and to reuse these for many days and years to come. For novelty, it is recommended that you try out different practices now and again that might be beneficial at different times and enhance your happiness perhaps in unexpected ways. This is one reason that challenges are included in the first appendix, to encourage you to explore and develop different angles for cultivating different aspects of happiness. This could support you in changing circumstances while keeping your brain stimulated, your curiosity piqued and your personal development growing.

If we can control our bodies then we can, to an extent, influence how we react and feel. For example: when we are more positive in our outlook and feel more upbeat, our bio-chemistry reflects this by producing feel-good chemicals. When we are negative and feel down, the bio-chemistry of stress infuses us. This also, obviously, directly influences our health, a clear link described by Dr Candace Pert, who explores the connection between emotions, bio-chemistry and immune-system function. She explains that positive emotions, such as happiness and its feel-good bio-chemistry, improve immune-system function; negative emotions, such as self-criticism and chronic stress, detract from health. When we feel happy, we also tend to be more resourceful, productive, effective, confident and creative; we feel life is more manageable and we can naturally be more resilient and bounce back quickly from setbacks. Yet, the feeling and tone of happiness can shift and change many times in our lives and even many times in a day depending on our circumstance, causing our bio-chemical levels to shift along with it.

What Are the Bio-chemicals of Happiness?

There are many bio-chemicals involved in our experience of happiness. The ones referred to in this book represent common chemicals associated with the various 'feeling tones' of happiness itself, or chemicals that support our ability to feel happy. They include:

- ✱ the hormone testosterone and the neurotransmitter dopamine, which boost our more extroverted happiness, along with our motivation to achieve in life;
- ✱ the neurotransmitter serotonin and the hormone oxytocin, which boost our quieter, more introverted and heartfelt happiness; and
- ✱ euphoric endorphins, which are hormones that also play their part in endurance and easing pain.

These bio-chemicals do not work in isolation from each other or from other chemicals produced in the body. The focus on one chemical at a time here is for the distinct feeling tone that we can come to associate with each and that can guide us to the kinds of behaviours that boost these various feeling tones.

5 Bio-chemicals of Happiness

1. Serotonin: Quiet Happiness and Self-worth

Serotonin is the bio-chemical most commonly associated with happiness. It is a neurotransmitter produced mainly in the gut, making it sensitive to our digestive health. It is also produced in the brain. Serotonin functions as a mood regulator and can influence both our good and bad moods. Serotonin is produced in response to light, explaining why sunshine tends to lift our spirits. This is due to a gland in the brain, the pineal gland, involved in the stimulation of serotonin and its nighttime partner melatonin. Researchers do not fully understand the function of the pineal gland. What we do know is that it is involved in producing and regulating some hormones, and that it contains photoreceptors, just like we have in our eyes. These photoreceptors are activated by light, producing serotonin to activate an awakened state, and melatonin in darkness to help us relax and fall asleep at night and regulate our sleep cycles. Serotonin has a close relationship with our calming parasympathetic nervous system in that when serotonin levels are healthy, we tend to feel more relaxed, sleep better at night and wake up feeling more refreshed in the morning.

The pineal gland has also been associated with our ability to feel connected with a spiritual realm. For example, pineal gland activity can be observed during dreaming and transcendental, hallucinatory or out-of-body experiences. Some speculate that naturally occuring DMT (dimethyltryptamine), colloquially referred to as *the spirit molecule* or *God molecule*, is produced by the pineal gland, while we sleep, perhaps explaining why our dreams can veer off into the unknown. It might also explain how we feel when deeply absorbed in meditation, prayer or any other way we might practise spirituality. Meditation can also increase serotonin levels, supporting the link between serotonin and our sense of spirituality or wholeness. With lots still to be verified about the pineal gland's role in general, it is agreed in spiritual circles that the pineal gland offers access to the highest source of ethereal energy available to humans.

Alongside the deeper possibility of serotonin boosting spirituality, on a much simpler level it provides feelings of quiet, deep-seated joy, grounded confidence, tranquility and inner peace, and is intimately involved in our sense of wellbeing. Serotonin has also been associated with self-esteem and is produced when we feel significant, realise our worth or reflect on what we have achieved in life. It is even produced when we imagine or remember times when we have experienced these feelings. Serotonin recedes when we feel lonely, insignificant or depressed.

Role in happiness: Builds deep reserves of energy, peace of mind and joy, supporting resilience and emotional stability.

❊ Quick Tips to Get the Serotonin Feeling ❊

- Smile for no reason and notice how your mood lifts and how warmth spreads through you.
- Remember a time when you felt good about yourself - perhaps a time you achieved something that you felt proud of.
- Find something to appreciate or feel grateful for in this moment.
- Bask in sunshine. You might also imagine becoming the sun or absorbing the sun into you so that the sun shines through you.
- Walk in nature, breathing in the fresh air and absorbing the sights, sounds and smells around you.
- Pause to appreciate beauty around you, in nature and in others.
- Savour the moment, such as pausing to take in a beautiful scene or appreciating kind words or eating slowly to enjoy your food more (this will help your digestion, too).

These are all examples of the warm, expansive, perhaps spiritual, feelings that serotonin can offer us.

2. Oxytocin: Meaningful Connection, Contribution and Belonging

Oxytocin is a hormone produced in the brain and discovered also in the heart. It is the invisible force that binds us to others and to our shared humanity. It is involved in feelings such as intimacy, love, trust and belonging. Oxytocin can have a soothing, calming and nurturing effect on us. This is because, as with serotonin, it has a close relationship with our calming parasympathetic nervous system.

Oxytocin has been referred to as a 'snuggle hormone' or 'cuddle hormone', as well as a 'hormone of love' and even a 'moral hormone' in the way that heartfelt connection can inspire moral behaviour. When we spend time with loved ones and when we are kind towards others, oxytocin is stimulated. When we make a meaningful contribution to society, it can also be stimulated. Touch is another way to naturally stimulate oxytocin in a matter of seconds (provided, of course, that touch is caring and that the recipient is open to receiving it). Oxytocin is a basic, vital need in healthy child development and continues to be essential to physical, emotional and mental health throughout our lives. It is also what allows us to feel empathy and compassion, and it can be an antidote to the stress hormone cortisol (which is explained below). Research has shown that those with high levels of oxytocin tend to rate their overall satisfaction in life as high.

Role in happiness: Builds intimacy, a sense of connection and belonging, as well as feelings of trust and love, which can tether us to our shared humanity.

❊ Quick Tips to Get the Oxytocin Feeling ❊

- Text or call a friend to say hello and ask how they are.
- Smile at somebody who looks friendly.
- Call up a happy memory with a loved one, or a fond memory of a dear pet.
- Practise random acts of kindness.
- Support, motivate and complement others.
- Place a hand on your chest for a sense of connection with yourself, through your heart.
- Reflect on how your work, or who you are, makes a meaningful difference to others.

The feelings derived from the above actions are all deeply nourishing oxytocin at work.

3. Dopamine: Creativity, Energy and Motivation

Dopamine is a neurotransmitter produced in the brain. It creates feelings such as excitement, anticipation, conviviality and enthusiasm, which can be really uplifting, motivating and energising. It is often called our 'motivation and reward molecule'. Dopamine drives our brain's reward system, fueling anticipation and motivating us to strive towards something exciting. Our reward system can be 'pinged' not only when we achieve big and exciting goals, but also when we get through all we want to in a day and tick off items on a to-do list. It could be as small as finishing the washing or larger like getting through spring cleaning or completing our exercise program for the day. Or it could be a more significant life goal like graduating from school or university, or winning a medal in sports. Whenever we feel like we have achieved something big or small, we get a dopamine boost or a 'Yes, I did it!' feeling of victory.

✳ Quick Tips to Get the Testosterone Feeling ✳

- Lengthen your spine to sit or stand tall, and hold your head up high. Take a deep breath to inflate your chest and then, when you exhale, keep your chest as open as feels comfortable. While taking a few more deep breaths in this upright position, feel inner strength, and perhaps determination, rising.
- Flex or tighten some muscles in your body for a boost to your sense of strength, willpower and determination.
- Power up your core strength by taking a few deep breaths into your belly, inflating your belly as you inhale and pressing your navel towards your spine as you exhale and then holding your belly slightly in towards your spine to help you stand or sit taller and feel more in control or stronger in yourself.

The feelings associated with these actions are all examples of the upstanding strength and personal power associated with testosterone.

5. Endorphins: Endurance and Euphoria

Endorphins are also not technically happy chemicals although they can cause us to feel happy or euphoric. Endorphins are actually stress bio-chemicals designed to numb pain and increase our endurance in times of need. They do so by interacting with the brain's opiate receptors to reduce our perception of pain with a naturally sedating effect. Endorphins can relieve both physical and psychological pain: they can help us through tough or traumatic accidents or injuries and emotional pain (such as depression, grief or trauma).

The endorphin experience can range from numbness to a 'second wind' of energy when we are tired and need to persevere. It can shower us in blissful euphoria after exertion (such as the 'runner's high') and help us go further and achieve more in life. This has won endorphins the nickname of 'endurance molecules', supporting our ability to push ourselves harder or go the extra mile in any arena such as at work or sport. In relation to physical exercise, any time we exert ourselves in a way that places stress on our bodies we can produce endorphins. This is why a challenging workout can feel so good. It is also true that the level of exertion required to produce endorphins differs from person to person and can relate to our level of fitness or familiarity with the form of exercise. For example, when we are new to certain forms of exercise, we can feel really elated afterwards (as well as perhaps physically stiff or sore). But when we become too familiar with our exercise routine and the level of challenge reduces while our fitness increases, our bodies produce less endorphins. At these times changing up our exercise routine or increasing intensity, repetitions or duration of exercise can increase our endorphin reward again. It is important to note that for optimal health we need to exercise within our range of capability and not push ourselves too hard and far, which can cause too much stress and have detrimental effects on our bodies and our health.

Laughter also releases endorphins; even the expectation of laughter can have the same effect. This is a good reason to attend comedy shows or watch funny films on TV, or see the lighter side of life when we can, for some welcome physical and emotional soothing. Music is also found to have a soothing, endorphin-stimulating effect on us, including when we listen or move to music and when we create music ourselves.

Role in happiness: Endorphins bring a euphoric high that helps us go further and achieve more in life, especially in stressful or really challenging situations. They also can provide emotional soothing.

Quick Tips to Get the Endorphin Feeling

- Exercise regularly in a way that provides sufficient physical challenge for an endorphin boost.
- Find opportunities to laugh (preferably with, and not at, others). Even smiling while exerting yourself can take the edge off pain and help you keep going for a bit longer.
- Put on some music, listen or move to it, or take part in creating music yourself, all potentially stimulating endorphin euphoria.
- Burn some oil in an oil burner or vaporiser, or spritz your rooms with essential oil mixes. The scent of lavender and vanilla have been associated with endorphin release and the activation of our calming, parasympathetic nervous system.

An Extrovert-Introvert Factor

For those who are more extroverted by nature, dopamine and testosterone can come more easily, bringing qualities such as confidence and enthusiasm. Extroverts can have a constant drive to go out into the world and seek the kind of stimulation that feeds their extroversion, like striving towards challenging and inspiring goals, or socialising. For introverts, testosterone or a dopamine rush can trigger anxiety or feeling overwhelmed.

The opposite is true about the quieter happy chemicals of serotonin and oxytocin that boost qualities such as inner peace and heartfelt connection. These can come naturally to introverts but can cause anxiety for extroverts who might not feel comfortable with quietude.

Luckily, with the practical exercises offered through the book, both introverts and extroverts can grow their ability to access and enjoy the full range of happy bio-chemistry. Introverts can develop their extroverted side for a boost in confidence, enthusiasm and sociability; and extroverts can develop their introverted side for a boost in mindfulness, connection and compassion. All together, inviting the full range of bio-chemicals allows for a well-rounded, sustainable experience of happiness in which we can achieve important goals and find deep enjoyment in the quieter side of life, too.

Endorphins are an exception to the extrovert-introvert factor because our bodies can be supported by endorphins no matter our personality traits. Endorphins can give us all a helping hand through emotional ups and downs and stressful or challenging times.

The Bio-chemical Blocking Your Happiness

Cortisol: Anxiety and Worry

The biggest offender in blocking happiness is cortisol, but only when stress levels are chronic. Cortisol is a steroid hormone produced in the adrenal glands. It is actually involved in many healthy functions of the body such as reducing inflammation, digestion and regulating blood pressure. When you are stressed, cortisol can also boost your energy to meet the demands of stress as well as restoring balance afterwards. But when stress is ongoing, cortisol levels remain high, with knock-on effects on your physical and psychological health. For example, chronic stress can have a detrimental effect on cardiovascular, digestive and immune system functioning and can cause inflammation.

Cortisol can prolong stress for hours, days or sometimes even years when our cortisol system is out of balance, keeping us trapped in some degree of stress response. This is often accompanied with chronic or frequent anxiety as cortisol levels can spike and sink more dramatically in relation to life experience than if our stress response system was in healthy balance. When cortisol levels drop too low it can also have the effect of draining our energy, creating low stress resilience, causing us to feel lethargic, depressed or burnt out, feeding into feelings such as desperation or despair and affecting our memory and concentration.

A study by scientists from Edinburgh and New York following 9/11 found that we can also pass on our stress tendencies to our children. In this study traumatised mothers who were pregnant while witnessing the collapse of the World Trade Center went on to give birth to babies who showed lower levels of cortisol, associated with chronic stress, by the time they were one year old. These mothers were also found to have low cortisol levels, considered to be a sign of post traumatic stress disorder (PTSD).

In survival terms, when a stress response is active there is no biological imperative to feel happy. The top priority is survival and finding our way to safety quickly. This is why cortisol blocks happiness.

✳ Quick Tip to Get the Cortisol, Stress-Hormone Feeling ✳

- Furrow your brow and notice how worry can quickly rise and affect your breathing. Early bio-feedback research made use of the frontalis muscle, which covers most of the forehead, as a way to detect shifts in emotional state. When we are calm, our forehead relaxes. When we worry, even slightly, our forehead muscles are activated.

If furrowing your brow has spiked your cortisol levels, hold a hand over your forehead for a few moments to encourage relaxation and to help you feel calmer and clearer. You can also stack a few of the short practices offered so far, such as righting your posture (from the introductory chapter) and bringing a small smile to your face or choosing any of the quick tips of this chapter to inspire your return to happiness.

CHAPTER 2
A HAPPY BALANCE

'Happiness is a journey, not a destination.'
ALFRED D. SOUZA

For happiness to be sustainable various feeling tones need to be balanced so that they can work together in a complementary way. In doing this we can come to realise that happiness is more like a journey than a destination. Every day we journey through a potentially wide range of ups and downs. Within qualities of happiness this range could include excited, enthusiastic and confident highs all the way through to grounded, quiet moments of inner peace and contentment. Our high moments would exhaust us if they were not balanced by wholesome, nourishing quiet times. Too much quietude could also be limiting in that we might not go out and make things happen for a truly fulfilling life. To be our best, our more extroverted qualities that feed happiness, such as ambitious striving (testosterone) and reward or novelty seeking (dopamine), must be complemented by our more introverted qualities, such as mindfulness (serotonin) and spending quality time with significant people and pets (oxytocin).

The ups and downs of our happy bio-chemistry can also represent different stages of life. For example there are years when we might feel motivated to reach new heights (dopamine and testosterone), like when we are starting a new business or taking a business or our personal life to a new level. These stages are helped by our more extroverted, outgoing qualities. Then there are times, like just after giving birth or as we mature and age, when we might want to slow down and be more introverted for a time (oxytocin and serotonin). No stage is the same for everyone. There are seventy year olds who finally choose to live their lives to the full and there are twenty year olds who believe in taking life as easy as possible. Life tends to fluctuate naturally and the more we listen to our natural rhythms, the more satisfied and happy we feel.

We might get this balancing act of happiness just right at times; at other times it might need refining. Knowing that we can intentionally orchestrate our happiness, however, can help us each become our own master conductors of happiness.

With this knowledge of how key bio-chemicals of happiness work together in 'happy balance', you are invited to reflect on how this might be playing out in your life, with the help of two brief self-assessments. The first invites you to reflect on what might be helpful to you at this point in time. The second invites you to consider what comes most naturally to you and your personality. There is a third assessment to follow in the next chapter, too, which focuses on the physical skills that correspond with our happy bio-chemistry.

Self-assessment №1

What Could Be Helpful to You at This Time?

Dopamine: Could you benefit from a dopamine boost to spark your inspiration, excitement, sense of adventure and fun, while increasing your energy levels and motivation too?

Oxytocin: Could you benefit from an oxytocin boost to feed your heart through quality time with the special people in your life, or some compassionate self-care, emotional soothing or some new way to make a meaningful contribution in the world?

Serotonin: Could you benefit from a serotonin boost through some rest, recuperation or reconnection with nature? This could involve some alone time to tune into yourself, like spending time in nature to help you feel more balanced and grounded.

Testosterone: Could you benefit from a testosterone boost to strengthen your confidence, determination, goal focus or willpower? This can help you stand tall, hold your head up high, go out into the world more confidently or stand up for what you believe in.

Endorphins: Could you benefit from some numbing or pain relief with the help of endorphins, to help you through a challenging time or to boost your endurance?

In happy balance: Or perhaps at this time, your energy feels just right and you might simply acknowledge this and feel grateful for it. Perhaps you can also reflect on the kind of day or week that you have had to create this sense of wellbeing. Usually it is a mix of feeling excited about life or having something exciting to look forward to (dopamine), feeling well rested and peaceful inside yourself (serotonin), having many friendly interactions with others (oxytocin), and feeling active, productive and on top of things (testosterone and dopamine – perhaps with the help of endorphins, too).

 What stands out for you as you read through this list? Keep this in mind as you carry out the next self-assessment (and the third in the next chapter, which can offer you further guidance).

 This brief self-assessment can be a way to get a quick read on your bio-chemical needs, at any point in time, as your moods, energy levels and circumstances evolve.

Self-assessment №2

What Comes Naturally to Your Personality?

Each of us can also have a personality that is stronger in particular areas, making it easy to access certain qualities but difficult to access others. With the help of the practical tools in this book, however, you can become more well-rounded, successful and happier even if your personality strengths remain the same. It is interesting to share this reflection process with someone who knows you well, who can probably point out in an instant your personality strengths.

Serotonin: Does it come naturally to you to think deeply about life, perhaps with a well-developed philosophical or spiritual side? Do you enjoy taking life slowly enough to savour your experiences, feel proud of your achievements, appreciate nature around you and feel grateful for what you have? Are you happy to spend time on your own and prefer to work and think alone, or at least have this time to feel prepared before collaborating with others?

Oxytocin: Does it come naturally to you to be an empath, really aware of, affected by and compassionate towards the feelings of others? Do you easily draw on the support of those around you and prefer one-on-one or small groups? Do you tend to be quiet and feeling-oriented?

Testosterone: Does it come naturally to you to be confident and assertive and feel really comforable in leadership roles? Do you think and work quickly and have little tolerance for emotionality?

Dopamine: Does it come naturally to you to be fun-loving, creative and motivating of others? Do words like enthusiastic, extroverted, excitable, highly social, collaborative and creative describe you well?

Endorphins: This is not so much a personality trait as a tendency towards certain kinds of behaviours that we can add to this assessment for the insight they can bring. Relating to endorphins, are you a person who enjoys pushing yourself hard, perhaps to new heights and ever-greater achievements? This could also be a testosterone trait, and it can have a flavour of endorphins, too, depending on how hard you push yourself and how much stress you might deliberately endure. Or is 'numbing out' something you feel you long for a lot in your life, which might be a sign of unresolved trauma? Maybe you arc a person who sees the lighter side of life, finding any reason for a laugh and perhaps enjoying making others laugh too?

How would you rate your personality in relation to these traits listed above? You are invited to list these traits from 1-5 in the table below, where 1 is the quality most dominant in you or most aligned with your natural ability, and 5 is the quality least dominant. Again, this exercise can make for interesting discussions with those you know well in your personal life or even at work.

1. _____

2. _____

3. _____

4. _____

5. _____

THE PHYSICAL SKILLS OF HAPPINESS

'The body has its own wisdom and ways of knowing, separate and distinct from that of the mind.'

JOHN KEHOE

There are particular physical skills that correspond with, and that can stimulate, the different chemicals of happiness. Grounding activities partner well with serotonin. Strength is a partner of testosterone. Fluidity, flexibility and agility are partners to dopamine. Warmheartedness is a partner to oxytocin. These skills can also help us with endurance or perseverance, which are partners to endorphins. These partnerships are introduced in this chapter. Then an entire section is dedicated to each of the skills that can develop our relationship with the specific chemicals, according to what would be most helpful at any given time.

This chapter also includes one more self-assessment – this time in relation to these physical skills. This is an opportunity to clarify your areas of strength and personal growth from a physical perspective. Then you are invited to make your way to the section of the book that provides information on the area you feel you could benefit most from develveloping at this time. This is also a book for you to return to many times over and for many years to come, as your needs and situations change and your happy balance tips one way or another.

The Physical Abilities That Make Up Your Happy Balance

Grounding

Serotonin's feelings of inner peace and perhaps a connection with something greater than ourselves is supported in our bodies by feeling physically balanced and grounded. Our relationship with gravity plays a role here. Gravity is the force that keeps us on the earth, preventing us from floating off into space. When we surrender our body weight into gravity, we feel more substantial and stable, literally *and* metaphorically. This can boost our sense of self-worth, offer an antidote for anxiety and help minimise depression, too. Ironically, when we feel more grounded and substantial, we can feel lighter or more spacious inside, such as the kind of experience that sitting in meditation can give us. This lightness can be encouraged any time we are upright, through good postural alignment. When we focus on our skeleton rather than our muscles to hold us upright, stacking and aligning our bones from the ground up, we possess a greater sense of balance. Then we experience a natural two-way pull as gravity grounds us downwards towards the centre of the earth, an experience we feel through our hips, legs and feet, while our sense of balance and levity flows upwards through our spine. The better our alignment, the better our sense of balance and postural ease and the more relaxed we can feel as we move through the world. Alignment is also conducive to using our energy well. If we are tense, our muscles have to work to maintain our uprightness and the more effort and energy it takes to move through life. This creates more wear and tear or burden on our bodies than necessary and can deplete our energy. Along with good postural alignment, tools for de-stressing are important, too, for maintaining the sense of being grounded, as well as getting sufficient rest, sleep and recuperation.

Brief Experience of Grounding

Physical points of grounding: Place both feet on the ground evenly and balance your weight over your hips. Feel the soles of your feet in contact with the ground (through your shoes if need be). You might like to imagine or feel an energy exchange between your feet and the ground as if the earth is energising you via your feet.

- *If you are standing,* shift your weight slightly back over your heels and relax your knees so that you can feel more grounded from hips down through heels (and ultimately towards the centre of the earth, which is the direction of gravity's pull).
- *If you are sitting,* along with grounding through your feet, also feel the weight of your upper legs and hips resting into your seat, which is in contact with the ground. If your hands are on your lap, also feel their weight as another point of contact with the pull of gravity.

Right your posture from the ground up: From this point, notice how you can right your posture from the ground up. If you are standing, you might press down into your feet and allow your body to unfold to comfortable uprightness. If you are sitting, you could press down into your hips and feel how the downward pressure into gravity helps your spine to find an upright position.

Loosen into the top of your neck: One final check is the very top of your neck, where your neck meets your skull. This area contains small bones that allow you to nod 'yes' or shake 'no'. When we get stuck in our thoughts or are focusing on a task for long periods, this part of our neck can lock or become tense. When this happens, it can feel as if you are holding your whole body up by your head. Or this upper neck tension can hold you back from fully experiencing the downward, nourishing and stabilising pull of gravity. To loosen up into your upper neck, take a few moments to nod and shake your head, and draw circles or other shapes in the air with the tip of your nose. Then feel how your head can almost float in its position at the top of your spine while you remain in touch with your grounding through your contact points with your seat and the ground.

Take 3–5 deep breaths, focusing on exhaling releasing into gravity: Maintaining this grounded, upright position, take 3–5 deep breaths through your nose, extending your exhalation for as long as you can. Further grounding is encouraged if you imagine letting go into gravity with each outbreath.

Quick grounding anytime reminder: Any time of the day you can remind yourself of your points of contact with the ground (feet, and underside of upper legs and hips if you are sitting, and perhaps hands if they rest in your lap or on your desk).

Strength

Testosterone's qualities of feeling strong in ourselves and empowered in life to achieve our goals is supported in our bodies by physical, muscular strength. When we feel strong physically it helps us

- Fluidity, flexibility and agility
- Warmheartedness

On the table below, 1 is what comes most naturally to you and 4 is what you feel you most need to develop at this time.

1. _____

2. _____

3. _____

4. _____

Client Story

Restoring a 'Happy Balance' at 50

Sybil was feeling emotionally overwhelmed, believing it was linked to her turning 50. The residue of old fear, pain, confusion, anger and low self-worth all seemed to be swirling inside her reminding her of her troubled past. She reached out to me for support. As Sybil spoke in our first session, I noticed that she had her right hand across her belly. I invited her to use this touch consciously by sliding her right hand up under her armpit with her palm against the side of her ribs, as if cradling her heart. I invited her to also bring her left hand across her chest to hold the outside of her right upper arm. This is a self-supportive hold originating in the acupressure system called Jin Shin Jyutsu. It can encourage a visceral sense of emotional containment. I call it an 'over-under' hug. My intention was to boost her oxytocin levels through the self-supportive touch, for some on-the-spot emotional soothing. I hoped this might also allow her to open up to her feelings in a way that felt safer.

Sybil shared that it helped her feel a bit stronger and more ready to explore her feelings, which she did while holding herself in this way until her arms tired of the position. Later in the session she even described the warmth and sense of emotional containment that resulted from the holding as magnificent, and we played with images like her skin as a royal velvet cloak that felt protective, sobering and strengthening when she needed it to be. This is a sign of serotonin-related qualities emerging, too. These qualities are linked with a higher sense of self-esteem and feeling more self-confident, while at the same time feeling more peaceful and safer inside ourselves.

Sybil shared how she could only connect with her skin in some parts of her body. With a history of abuse, as Sybil had experienced, it is possible to sever awareness of certain parts of our body in order to avoid triggering old feelings, or to numb pain. But claiming back more of her skin and her body felt of the utmost importance to Sybil now. She wanted to claim her right to live more fully. The more we grow our sense of occupying or living inside of our bodies, the more substantial we feel. These feelings are also associated with serotonin's quiet self-confidence, deeply rooted in feeling grounded and substantial, helping us feel more emotionally stable and resilient.

During our work together that spanned a number of sessions Sybil shared details of her painful past, shed some tears, felt scared and angry at times and found her way to some laughter too and through it all was able to feel held and supported. This was facilitated by my therapeutic attentiveness and by her own hands at important moments too.

We also spoke about 50 being an age of starting to think about our life legacy. In this we began to organically call on dopamine qualities with the question of what might make life feel worth living. It could be sharing her talents more than before, or feeling more comfortable and confident in who she was and what she might want to achieve in life. When conversations meander in this direction it can bring a sparkle to the eyes, an animation to the face and a tendency to gesticulate more expressively. This is a sign of dopamine levels rising, waking up a sense of possibility, inspiration or excitement. It also can boost a sense of freedom and open us to being more adventurous and risk-taking.

Sybil had a passion for writing that she had not pursued. She shared about an idea that she had been thinking about for writing a novel inspired by themes from her own life. Writing her novel felt important at this time to help her rewrite her life story in a way that felt empowering. From a bio-chemical perspective this again represented a boost to her dopamine levels through the new and positive way of portraying her history. It also represented a boost to her sense of personal strength and determination to experience life differently (testosterone) as well as nourishing her self-esteem (serotonin) that was beginning to blossom from deep inside her.

Towards the end of this piece of work she proclaimed: 'This is Sybil. Why haven't I lived like this before? I want to now . . .' Since then Sybil still finds herself challenged and scared at times and her excitement and energy for her new life after 50 is palpable, carrying her through fearful moments. Along with the help of daily ways to top up on and balance the bio-chemistry that she needs, Sybil is living into a deeper sense of happiness than she has ever experienced before.

CHAPTER 4

GROUNDING TECHNIQUES AND SUPPORTING RESILIENCE

'Feeling rooted in the earth is soothing to the body, and it is our connection to the earth that gives us our most basic sense of belonging, home, resilience, and safety.'

JESSICA MOORE

Grounding is the art of drawing on the earth's gravitational force as a valuable resource. On earth, gravity gives weight or mass to objects, including our sense of ourselves, which can feel more substantial when we are grounded. Natural outcomes of being grounded include a calm and stable experience of joy from the inside out, greater appreciation of things around us, enhanced mental clarity and presence, and increased resilience during life's ups and downs. These are all qualities associated with healthy serotonin levels. One of the ways that grounding works is by releasing nervous-system energy in the same way that a grounding cord gives a channel for electricity to discharge safely. When we feel stressed or emotional, grounding can give the feeling of stress draining out of us, down into the earth, freeing our minds to think more clearly and creatively.

Grounding can offer a primal sense of safety in body and mind. You might equate this to the feeling of being a child or a baby, safe in your parent's arms, completely relaxed in their care. Grounding practices can also be a remedy if consistent loving care was lacking from your caregivers. It can offer your nervous systems a way to release pent-up tensions, feel supported from the ground up or, if you like, supported by Mother Earth. You might also become more receptive to your surroundings via your five senses of sight, touch, sound, taste and smell and your sixth gut or intuitive sense, too.

You can increase your sense of grounding in two ways:

- Being grounded and present in your body
- Feeling connected to the earth

Removing your shoes and being in physical contact with grass, sand or rocks, and spending time in nature are powerful ways to increase your sense of grounding and you can draw on grounding and centring through the body anywhere and any time. Grounding can make a big difference to our state of mind and resilience while feeding a calm and stable sense of happiness.

How do you know when you are not grounded? Are you over-thinking, worrying or perhaps obsessing about something? Are you feeling scattered and easily distracted? Or might you feel a bit spaced out?

If the answer is yes to any of these, then you might benefit from a grounding technique to help you be more present, recharge your energy, think more clearly and feel stronger and more stable in yourself.

Grounding in Your Body

Grounding in your body amplifies sensory awareness (sight, sound, taste, smell, touch and intuitive or gut sensing). This can enhance your sense of presence and your ability to appreciate or savour each moment more fully. It can also enhance your sense of being in touch with yourself in an authentic kind of way because of the heightened sensory awareness. Along with this it is possible to experience your inner world as expansive, as if you are able to connect with something greater than yourself. This can feel inspiring, perhaps in a spiritual kind of way.

When we are familiar with grounding techniques we can choose to ground ourselves on the spot, anywhere and any time, shifting awareness from mind into body. This can have an almost instant calming effect because it activates our parasympathetic nervous system, specifically the vagus nerve that plays a central role in our deep-rooted experience of happiness.

6 Techniques for On-the-spot Grounding

You are invited to experiment with the following techniques and choose what works best for you.

1. **Find your centre of balance:** Place your feet evenly on the ground. If you are sitting, sit evenly over your hips so that you feel more balanced. Allow your posture to naturally adjust to being more upright and open as you feel into your body's centre of gravity. Take 2–3 deep breaths into this more centred, balanced and grounded position before returning to your day.

2. **Place a hand on the crown of your head:** This can feel like placing a lid on your thinking, instantly helping you to feel more grounded in your body, instead, and present in the moment. This action can also help when you are feeling light-headed. Hold for as briefly or long as you need.

3. **Release your breath:** Breathe in through your nose for a mental count of 4, hold for a count of 6 or 7, blow the air out slowly through your mouth for 7 or 8. Repeat 3 times. This breathing technique can be helpful to release fear, worry or anxiety. As you slowly breathe out it can be helpful to imagine energy releasing out with your breath as well as down through your belly, legs and feet and on deep down into the earth. Finish by taking a few moments to notice how your feet feel: they might feel a bit tingly with your grounding. If something has been on your mind, it can be interesting from this grounded perspective to ask yourself: 'How can I see things differently now?' Then notice what might come to mind.

4. **Hang forwards over slightly bent legs:** This can be done at any time of day and will help you to release tension and lengthen out your spine. To move into the position, start by standing with feet hip distance apart and parallel with knees a little bent. Shift your weight back slightly over your heels for stability as you lower your head and gradually roll down your spine, moving your head down towards the ground until your body, from hips to fingertips, is hanging forward over your legs in a position that feels comfortable. Check that your weight is back slightly over your heels for maximum grounding effect. Hold the position for 5 breaths, or longer if you wish. Then slowly unfold your body to upright, keeping your legs slightly bent as you make your way back. Repeat one or two more times if you wish.

5. **Gentle bounce while standing:** In a standing position, with feet flat on the ground, bounce gently into your knees, encouraging a feeling of weight. This can add some buoyancy to your grounding, perhaps adding a spring to your step. When you return to standing, keep your knees unlocked so that you can move about more freely and stay more in touch with the ground beneath you.

6. **'Vuuu' or 'Aum' sound:** On a long exhalation, make a 'Vuuuuu' sound (as in 'Vooooo') to support your feeling physically calmer and mentally clearer. It can be helpful to imagine your 'Vuuu' sound as a foghorn to amplify the grounding effect. The 'Vuuu' sound is inspired by the work of trauma expert Dr Peter Levine, who uses it to help clients feel more grounded in their bodies in order to increase their receptivity to trauma therapy. It works because extended exhalations stimulate our parasympathetic, calming nervous system. Added to this, different sounds tend to resonate in different parts of the body. An 'Oooo' sound tends to resonate low down in the belly and pelvic bowl, amplifying the grounding effect. This is as compared with other sounds like singing 'Aaah' that can also be relaxing but not quite as grounding because it tends to resonate higher up in the chest and throat areas. You might try out different sounds to explore where they resonate in your body. An 'Aum' or 'Om' sound on a long exhalation can also have a calming and grounding effect as it resonates in the belly area. Repeat the 'Vuuuu' or 'Aum' sound 3 times then pause to take note of how your body feels. This practice can be added to a morning routine or used during your commute to work (such as in the car or quietly on the train) or any time you feel you could benefit from this quick reset to a more grounded frequency.

Feeling Connected to the Earth, or *Earthing*

Earthing can be seen as the ultimate form of grounding. It refers to the kind of grounding facilitated by direct skin contact with the earth, such as when we walk barefoot on grass, sand or rocks or getting down on our hands and knees to do some gardening. It is believed that being in direct contact with the earth allows for the transfer of earth's free electrons from the ground into the body. Benefits of at least 20 minutes of direct contact with the earth or nature include better sleep, reduced pain and inflammation, increased resilience, normalisation of daily cortisol rhythms to help us with stress management, reduced anxiety, improved mental health and increased serotonin levels, to boost our sense of vitality. One applied example of this can be seen in gardening projects springing up all over the world in prisons and mental health facilities, for the positive effects they have on mental health.

Ideas for Topping Up Your *Earthing* Reserves

This is as easy as taking off your shoes and socks and spending time outside whenever you get a chance. It could involve spending time in botanical gardens, on the beach, going on mountain or forest walks, sitting by a rocky stream, or whatever you have access to, to build up your reserves. Any natural surface can do the trick. Besides Earthing, spending time barefoot also helps to keep your feet more pliable and flexible. I also find it nourishing to pause and appreciate nature around me whenever I can, such as including natural touches in my home – a vase of flowers or plants or wooden furniture.

What's your favourite way of topping up your *Earthing* reserves?

Resilience Versus Burn-out

Resilience is your capacity to recover from adversity or stress and respond with flexibility and adaptability. Life experience and your basic temperament can all influence how resilient you are, but it is also a skill that you can develop. Grounding serves a particular role in resilience by replenishing your energy reserves and giving you greater stability as you navigate life's ups and downs. Grounding can serve like internal cushioning, helping you to absorb and bounce back from life's knocks as memory foam does for comfortable beds and pillows.

When your grounding, or internal cushioning, is well established, it can keep you calmer, clearer, more mindful and resilient as you move through life. You might notice that your breathing is generally easier, you feel naturally happy or content, you are able to take life's ups and downs in your stride, and you can address challenges more intelligently and resourcefully. Compare this with when you feel really worn out at the end of a busy day or week, or when you're overstretched. These are the times you might tend to be irritable, jumpy and quick to lose your temper at every little annoyance. Along with this you might also struggle to concentrate or perform at your best and perhaps find that your willpower wanes, making you more prone to unhealthy choices. You can treat these times as invitations to top up on grounding in your favourite ways.

Resilience can be helped by other bio-chemicals too. Oxytocin's gentle nurturing and mutual support has an important part to play in helping us recover emotionally from setbacks. Bouncing back with positivity and new, motivating vision can also serve a crucial role, which is the realm of dopamine. There are also times when for our resilience we need to rise above challenges and be strong or courageous, helped by testosterone.

Burn-out happens when resilience is chronically depleted affecting our ability to function productively and rebound from stress. Energy levels can be very low, leading us perhaps to rely on caffeine or medication to boost them. Due to its increasing prevalence, in May 2019, for the first time in history, burn-out was included in the International Classification of Diseases (ICD-11). It has been referred to as an 'occupational phenomenon'. However, it is also possible to experience burn-out in other contexts, where responsibilities and commitments become too much to bear, such as parenting or when confronting really challenging personal situations such as illness or loss.

From a physiological point of view, burn-out points to adrenal fatigue from prolonged stress, exertion, or feeling chronically over-extended. In the most serious cases this state can be life-threatening, although the burn-out mostly experienced from overwork is usually just a serious cry for help and change.

It is important to find the right remedy to fit the root cause of burn-out so that our resilience reserves can be replenished. In a personal context it might be that we need more support or courage to make necessary changes or vision to inspire us. In a professional context it could be a relationship dynamic in the workplace, an excessively heavy workload, job insecurity or something to do with the business as a whole. There is also a societal or global economic context that work-related burn-out can be placed in where the global work culture, particularly in corporate settings, places very high demands on individuals and on the business as a whole to stay relevant and afloat in our competitive, fast-paced times. It is also becoming clearer that when companies invest in the wellness of their employees it boosts morale and has a positive impact on job performance, healthy competitiveness and profitability. In this way organisational and employee resilience can both be cushioned to promote mutual happiness and success.

Client Story

From Burn-out to Good Leadership with the Support of Grounding

Sarah was a 42-year-old senior manager in a globally listed company. She was promoted into this position on the merit of her track record of excellent performance in her previous roles in the same company. A competent team was assembled under her. All team members were experienced in the business, complementing each other with different areas of strength and specialisation.

By the time I was called in to provide her with executive coaching, one year into her stepping into her leadership role, Sarah was practically in tears from chronic stress to the point of describing herself as 'burnt out'. Her team had also been underperforming, which was of concern to both her and the business.

Sarah spoke of feeling like she always worked the hardest and how she believed that, under pressure (which was regularly), she was the only one who could get the job done properly. Playing into this was Sarah's tendency to micro-manage her team members, often completing their work for time-sensitive tasks and working extra long hours to accomplish this. Sarah felt physically drained by it all and like she could not cope anymore.

Through our conversations Sarah realised that she needed to step back from micro-management as it was clearly interfering with her team members performing to their peak. She shared how, throughout her life, she had always turned to self-sufficiency and self-reliance under pressure. Professionally it had allowed her to excel. Now it was showing up as an area for growth in her leadership. She needed to learn to share and delegate responsibility, as well as to motivate and develop her team to perform at its best. In this she needed to learn how to conserve her own energy as a leader so that she could focus on the bigger picture and strategic thinking.

Grounding techniques made a significant difference for Sarah. As a regular practice, Sarah found it helpful to pause now and again through the day and use a physical reminder to ground. She liked the practice of centring her body by placing her two feet evenly on the ground and her two hips evenly on her seat if she was seated. She came to notice an unconscious habit of standing more on her left foot with her right foot slightly out to the side, resting with only toes on the ground as if always ready to move on to the next thing. She found this revealing of her tendency to always feel in a rush. Even though she found it exhilirating to be super productive, she could see how this style of operating was not helpful to those whom she worked with who found it difficult to engage with her as well as not good for her own health, as she walked around with high levels of chronic tension. As soon as she would notice herself standing more over one foot, she would immediately place both feet evenly on the ground and establish a more centred standing position before carrying on with what she was doing. In just a couple of seconds she described how this would shift her to feeling more present and mentally clearer. She also came to realise that she could function efficiently without needing to rush. Her team and colleagues really appreciated her greater presence and attunement to them too. As part of this process Sarah did also need to grapple with her belief that nobody else could do the job as well as she could and let go of her need to be in control of everything, which clearly had not been working.

With two feet on the ground, she would often add a few deep breaths and carry out a quick body scan to release tension and invite herself to surrender into gravity. If needed Sarah would also take a moment to ask herself what she needed to let go of in that moment, which was often the need for everything to be perfect. These interventions could take just a couple of minutes and would leave her feeling calmer and clearer.

Soon after our work began, Sarah decided to enrol in a meditation course to enhance her ability to live in a more grounded and present way. She credits a daily 20-minute meditation practice, which she enjoyed first thing in the morning, for really consolidating her more mature leadership style. Along with meditation, she also became more disciplined about not working after hours except in emergency situations and instead prioritised a good night's sleep which also felt very supportive of a more relaxed and happier frame of mind. In the work context Sarah realised she also wanted more mentorship to support her leadership position, which was provided along with HR support for team development to assist with her team's success.

Six months later her team's performance had improved dramatically and Sarah enjoyed her leadership role much more than before. She also felt generally happier as she discovered many gifts in taking life a bit slower and living in a more relaxed and grounded way. Gifts included an increased sense of wellbeing, improved quality of her relationships and feeling like she was enjoying life more.

About Meditation

Sitting meditation invites you to hold a comfortable, upright and grounded sitting position for a period of time while focusing the mind (such as by observing breathing or body sensations). The intention is not to stop your thoughts, but rather to discover, as Deepak Chopra refers to it, 'The quiet that is already there, buried under the thousands of thoughts the average person thinks every day.' One natural outcome is grounding simply from the endurance of stillness. Studies have found that meditation also influences our bio-chemistry in many ways, including our serotonin levels. For example, studies testing urine samples for signs of serotonin breakdown have been carried out on participants pre- and post-meditation. Serotonin levels were found to rise significantly following meditation. In one such study, by Bujatti and Biederer, focusing on transcendental meditation, the urine samples of participants who maintained a regular meditation practice was compared with non-meditators. The regular meditators showed higher serotonin levels than non-meditators in general, and the difference in serotonin levels rose even higher directly following a single meditation session. These are some of the ways in which meditation can benefit us:

It reduces fear: Low serotonin levels are often linked to depression, but there is also a connection between serotonin and fear. When a person experiences serotonin deficiency they might also have a higher fear response and be more prone to panic attacks. Meditation and living in a more grounded way can buffer you against fear and chronic anxiety, while building your internal reserves of emotional resilience.

It boosts immunity: Our immune system can also benefit. For example, in a Japanese study by Tamiguchi, Hirokawa, Tsuchiya and Kawakami, it was shown that 10 minutes of relaxation training (meditation can be a form of this) increases salivary immune system markers in female Japanese medical workers. This shows us that living in a more grounded, relaxed way is good for our health, helping to buffer us against the common cold, or at least potentially reducing the symptoms of our ailments and helping us recover more quickly.

It's more effective than simply relaxing: Compared with sitting and relaxing, as we might do lounging on the couch, studies show that the focused practices used in meditation, such as observing breathing, body sensations or the repetition of particular words, have far greater effectiveness on relaxation. For example, one study through Carnegie Mellon University comparing simple relaxation with meditation found that meditation had significantly greater effect on stress resilience and on optimising brain connectivity for better attentiveness and for engaging the executive control regions of our brain. This study also pointed to anti-inflammatory effects and improved immune-system functioning benefits.

There are many meditation techniques to choose from. If you are looking for a practice, you might experiment with a course or class on offer in your area. Or you can use the short meditation practice included at the end of the grounding workout in this book.

*Helpful Workout Recommendation
(In the workout section at the end of this book)
GROUNDING WORKOUT WITH SHORT MEDITATION

CHAPTER 5

SLEEP SUPPORT

*'Sleep that knits up the ravelled sleeve of care . . .
balm of hurt minds, great nature's second course.
Chief nourisher in life's feast.'*

WILLIAM SHAKESPEARE, *MACBETH*

This is your time to yawn and get ready for a relaxing read. It is an opportunity to reflect on and explore supportive strategies that might help the quality of your sleep so that you wake up feeling fresh for your day. Sleep is included in the section on grounding because it is one of the biggest contributors to how naturally grounded we feel. Sleep draws on serotonin's night-time partner, melatonin. Sleep also boosts other bio-chemical levels such as our calming acetylcholine and GABA (gamma-aminobutyric acid) levels as well as our regenerative HGH (human growth hormone) levels.

To help you reap these benefits, this chapter offers calming physical practices that you might try, to help you wind down and quiet your mind before bed. There are also on-the-spot techniques for when you are lying in bed that can help you fall asleep or return to sleep peacefully. Napping during the day is also touched on for the value it can add.

increasing the likelihood of feeling overwhelmed by stress and making us more irritable and emotionally sensitive in our relationships.

For all these reasons, it is a good idea to prioritise a good night's sleep.

How Much is Enough Sleep?

- ❄ Babies need the most sleep, averaging around 14–18 hours a day in increments.
- ❄ Toddlers of 1 to 2 years old need approximately 12–14 hours, which includes daily napping.
- ❄ Children 3–5 years need about 11–13 hours of sleep per night.
- ❄ By school-going age, children aged 6–13 years ideally should get 9–12 hours of sleep per night.
- ❄ Teenagers 14 years and up ideally need 8–10 hours of sleep per night.
- ❄ The ideal benchmark for adults is 7–8 hours of sleep per night.
- ❄ From about 60, many people tend to sleep fewer hours and often less deeply.

Different people can get away with different amounts of sleep, of course, but less than five hours of sleep per night on a regular basis is too little for optimal physical, emotional and mental functioning for adults. It is also found that a regular sleep routine of going to bed and rising at around the same time every day is better for optimal brain functioning and health than a varied sleep pattern. We can bounce back from a break from the normal routine now and again, like when we might go out or work late at night. But try to get back to your regular routine as quickly as possible.

It can happen (hopefully not often) that you lie awake for some time during the night. At these times it is recommended to stay lying down with your eyes closed for as long as you can as even just lying down is a break for your body and brain from the day, allowing your body to lightly go on with its recuperation functions. If anxiety plagues you then soothing yourself, such as using one of the techniques offered later in this chapter for quieting and soothing mind and body while lying down, can help you to relax and rest. Then you might use the time to meditate while lying down with any technique you might prefer or allow your mind to wander aimlessly – the key is doing your best not to get hooked into triggering feelings so as to remain relaxed. You might also need to address an issue that is on your mind and keeping you awake at night, in which case you can prioritise this in the daytime.

Napping

It is possible to top up on sleep with naps during the day. In this way you can make up some of your sleep requirement and top up your energy levels. Benefits of daytime naps can include increase in alertness, creativity, stamina, accuracy and stress resilience. Naps can also brighten your mood and boost your memory.

A 10–20 minute nap can have a restorative effect. Even better, especially when you have not slept enough at night, is a 60–90 minute siesta, which can recharge your energy and reboot both your mental processing and optimism. There is also some benefit to be had from a very short powernap, such as during the course of a busy work day. This could involve shutting your eyes, resting your head back on your seat and allowing your brain to switch off for as little as 2–5 minutes (if this is all you can manage). Setting an alarm for the time you have is advised, so that you can relax into the nap more fully. Stress levels calm because any time you relax completely, your body produces fewer stress hormones like cortisol and adrenaline. Even if short, a nap can be enough to help you through your day.

Sleep Support Practices

- 3 techniques to quiet and soothe mind and body while lying down.
- Child's pose before bed, to help you relax.
- Ice your head if you really struggle to fall asleep.

Try the following 3 techniques and choose the one that might work best for you.

1. Slowed-down breathing : This is a gentle breathing practice to help with relaxation. Close your eyes and breathe entirely through your nose if you can. Take 3–5 even breaths (or more if you like), slowing down your inhalation and exhalation. You might start by breathing in for a count of 3 and out for 3. Then in for 4, out for 4. Then in for 5, out for 5. If you wish, continue increasing the length of each breath; or, if 5 is your maximum count, repeat to that maximum count for another 2–3 breaths. Then return to your natural breathing and notice how your body feels for a moment before letting go into sleep.

2. Release breathing: This is a stronger practice for releasing tension and inducing relaxation towards better sleep. With eyes closed, inhale quietly through your nose for a count of 4 seconds.

Hold for 7 seconds. Then slowly blow your breath out through your mouth for a count of 7–8 seconds. Imagine releasing the energy of your day as you blow out each exhalation. Repeat as many times as you need to feel ready for sleep.

3. Self-supportive hold sequence: This can be added on to the breathing practice of your choice (above) or used on its own to soothe you into a peaceful night's sleep. Hold each position for about 20–30 seconds, or as long as you like before moving on to the next position.

- ✵ Hold your hands to the sides of your head, with fingers wrapped over the top of your head.
- ✵ Hold the base of your skull with one hand (any hand) to where your neck meets your head and place the other hand over your forehead.
- ✵ Keep the one hand on your forehead and move the other hand to your chest.
- ✵ Keep the hand on your chest and move the other hand to your lower belly, finding the place that feels best for you, below your navel.
- ✵ Place both hands flat on your thighs just below your hips or as far down as you can reach, to bring warmth to your legs.
- ✵ End with one hand (any hand) holding behind your neck, cradling the base of your head, and the other hand placed on your chest for a few more soothing breaths to connect your head and heart. Then move into your favourite sleeping position for a wonderful sleep.

*Helpful Workout Recommendation
(In the workout section at the end of this book)
BEDTIME WORKOUT FOR UNWINDING TOWARDS PEACEFUL SLEEP

Child's Pose Before Bed, to Help You Relax

If you only have time for just one relaxation pose before bed, the child's pose is a good one to choose. You can move into a child's pose on a comfortable (perhaps carpeted) surface and place your forehead on the ground. Take a few moments to find the most comfortable position for your arms. This might be with your lower arms resting along the ground, at your sides, with shoulders relaxed over your knees. Or you might prefer to extend your arms ahead of you, alongside your head with palms and elbows resting on the ground. Once you find your most comfortable position, relax there for a few quiet minutes, inviting your body and mind to let go. Turn inwards and quiet down in preparation for sleep.

Ice Your Head if you Really Struggle to Fall Asleep

It is known that our calming parasympathetic nervous system and its central vagus nerve are stimulated by the cold. Focusing this cooling effect on the front area of your brain, just behind your forehead, has been recognised as helpful with sleep. This is the brain area active when our minds are busy with thinking. The cooling effect on the brain, called cerebral hypothermia, has been found to reduce activity in this brain area and help lull us to sleep.

To achieve this, lie down when you are ready for sleep and place an icepack wrapped in a small soft towel over your forehead. If it is a home-made ice pack, you could keep it on to help quiet and slow down your mind before sleep and then remove it when you feel ready. Or you might be able to find an ice cap that can serve the purpose even better. An ice cap is the mechanism used in a pioneering study led by sleep expert Dr Eric Nofzinger. It is designed to cool the brain during sleep, resulting in a reduction in metabolism in the brain's frontal cortex associated with restorative sleep. With insomnia, an increase in metabolism is seen in this brain region, which is what the cooling cap targets. The caps use circulating water to keep the brain cool while sleeping, helping insomniacs fall asleep quickly and stay asleep as long as people without insomnia. Ice caps are becoming more available although you might need to look online or ask at your local health store, pharmacy or sleep institute to get hold of one.

*Helpful Workout Recommendation

(In the workout section at the end of this book)

BEDTIME WORKOUT FOR UNWINDING TOWARDS PEACEFUL SLEEP

CHAPTER 6
BOOSTING STRENGTH AND CONFIDENCE

*'At the center of your being you have the answer;
you know who you are and you know what you want.'*

LAO TZU

In September 2019, I witnessed a protest while living in South Africa. It had so many in the country fired up. It was a week when it was revealed that yet more women had fallen victim to violence at the hands of criminal men. It was a week where hundreds of people poured down to protest in front of parliament, all dressed in black and calling on the government to step up and do more to stop the scourge of gender-based violence. It was a week where even walking in the local shopping mall you could see many shop assistants and civilians with 'Enough!' written in black across their cheeks and arms. Shock waves and fervour seemed to spread far and wide as people stood tall and strong, individually and in solidarity with each other.

During this week I saw a client in tears, affected by these events. Also feeling fired up, her sentiment had fuelled a personal realisation that enough was enough in her life too – specifically applying to her work. Enough was enough for being overlooked for promotion. Enough was enough for playing small and nice about it. Enough was enough of acting like everything was OK.

When you relax your arms after the stretch, keep up with breathing into your chest area and hold your head up high to maintain a posture of greater confidence.

2. Stand in a Posture of Strength and Authority

When we stand tall, hold our heads up high and make our bodies look and feel bigger and stronger, it can lead us to feeling stronger and more confident in ourselves. Add a few deep breaths and feel your feet well grounded and your posture can help you transform feeling emotionally overwhelmed to new determination, or feeling timid to feeling more confident or mental confusion to a sense of greater clarity and resolve.

3. Flex or Tighten Your Muscles

Flexing muscles is a classic and primitive way to show strength. One study in 2011 from the universities of Singapore and Chicago titled *From Firm Muscles to Firm Willpower* explored this link between flexing or tightening muscles and perseverance. The study made a connection between muscle tightening and deliberately harnessing willpower or self-regulation towards achieving long-term goals. Participants were asked to tighten muscles somewhere in their bodies, such as in their hands, legs, gluteals or biceps, while exposed to a circumstance that required self-control: drinking a bad-tasting vinegar drink, resisting eating tempting but unhealthy foods, and immersing hands in a bucket of ice. The act of tightening muscles was found to strengthen their willpower or determination to avoid temptation, or to resist showing strain. To try this out for yourself, you could pick any muscle group to tighten and release, perhaps repeating a few times to explore how your determination and perseverance might be boosted to serve the important goals that promote your happiness. You can even do so inconspicuously, making it a readily available practice no matter where you might be. But be sure to release your muscles afterwards to avoid building up too much tension.

4. Engage Your Core Muscles

Naturally this is helped if you have a regular practice to strengthen your core and for a quick core trick try balancing on one leg and holding still for as long as you can. Repeat on the other leg. Or simply hold in your belly slightly, which encourages you to breathe and expand into your chest area, linked with feeling more confident. In general, core strength sends an empowering message from gut to brain, helping us to feel more in control.

5. Lift Weights

This can boost your sense of strength as well as charging up your emotional strength and your sense of being able to cope or rise to meet the challenge. You might use a pair of dumbbells if you have them, or a pair of full 2-litre milk bottles (one in each hand) that you could raise to shoulder height with arms bent and then as best you can press them up high above your head, then lower back down and repeat a few times. You could achieve the same outcome by carrying your shopping bags or anything else that reminds you of your physical strength. Just take care to remain within your capability and not push yourself too far, so as to avoid injury. In general, lifting weights is an excellent way to build strength and it can be wise to consult with a fitness expert to get you started in a way that works best and most safely for your body and capability.

*Helpful Workout Recommendation
(In the workout section at the end of this book)
STRENGTH WORKOUT

her home country. The centring practice has since became a tool that she draws upon any time she needs a boost to her strength and mental clarity. She also came to realise that the need for her support system is not a weakness; rather, it can now be a conscious choice as to how she chooses to live her life.

A Personal Bubble for Self-care and Inclusivity

A personal bubble is a visualisation in which we delineate our personal space for the sake of emotional containment and mental clarity. When I am about to give a presentation and I can see the audience in front of me, I like to take a moment to expand my personal bubble so that my energy feels like it grows to be able to touch each person in the room. On the other hand, a client of mine whose work is all about giving to others through corporate coaching, prefers to visualise her personal bubble just for herself, as a way to contain and nourish her own energy that can easily become scattered around others. This is because by nature she is highly sensitive to others' feelings, describing her personal boundary as 'porous'. So a practice of visualising and strengthening her sense of her personal boundary for self-care purposes works really well for her.

Here are 5 ways to apply a personal bubble visualisation. Try them out to discover how they might work for you.

1. Imagine a Bubble Around You

First imagine a bubble surrounding your body, then notice how close or far it needs to be for you to feel just right in this moment. There are times you might require more self-containment and times you might feel more expansive with your energy. There is no right or wrong.

2. Clear Your Personal Bubble

If you feel stressed, notice if anything or anyone feels as if they are inside of your personal bubble with you – probably linked with something that's been on your mind. Acknowledge who and what this might be and kindly ask each one to leave so that your space can be yours. They can wait outside of your bubble so that you can be more present both with them and with yourself.

3. Centre and Relax in Your Personal Bubble

This combines a centring practice with a gentle breathing practice to increase your sense of comfort and relaxation inside of your bubble. After visualising your personal bubble, find your centre in your favourite way (refer to centing options). Then take a few deep breaths. Imagine your breath flowing up your back on inhalation and down your front on exhalation. Feel strength in the inhalation and allow the front of your body to soften and relax on exhalation. Try smiling while you do this, perhaps helped by thinking of someone who makes you happy.

4. Expand Your Bubble for Your Awareness to be More Inclusive of Others or Your Surroundings

To do this, look out to the corners of the room that you are in or take in your surroundings more fully if you are outside. If you are in front of a group that you are about to present to, allow your awareness to expand to include the whole group. Play with expanding your bubble to be able to touch and include the whole group and notice how your presence grows in the process. Smile, and imagine this happiness spreading outwards too, to fill your whole bubble and spread outwards into the room or space that you are in. Experiment with what might work best for you.

5. Build Your Physical Sense of Your Personal Boundary

Using physical movement you can support your sense of strength and personal boundary, linked with qualities like self-confidence and the ability to say 'No'. This can support personal integrity and ultimately happiness at times when this kind of strength boost is needed, such as in preparation for dealing with a challenging person. The physical movement involves taking even just a few minutes to practise physically delineating a boundary around you with your hands. You might outline the perimeter of your bubble with the palms of your hands, delineating front, sides, top, bottom and back of your personal space bubble.

Powering Up With Breath

'If there is any human super power, it's breathing. Not only is it the strongest link between life and death, it gives us the power to change the way we think, feel and move.'

DANA SANTOS

Breath is life. It is with us from our first breath after birth all the way through to our last breath when life withdraws from our body. Breath is also associated with our life force or spirit. For example, in the yogic tradition, breath is referred to as *prana,* understood as both breath and life force or subtle, vital energy that animates us and can connect us with our spiritual nature. In Latin, the word *spiritus* refers to both spirit and breath as well as to the qualities of courage and vigour. These are just a few of many examples of the breath-spirit connection and how we breathe more fully and steadily to facilitate inspiration and life.

Breathing is unique in our physiology in that it is both automatic and consciously controlled. When we ignore it, breathing continues all on its own to keep us alive day and night. When we control it deliberately, or bring our awareness to our breathing, we can harness our breathing for various purposes such as calming us down when we are worked up or building up our energy when we feel flat.

6 Breathing Practices That Can Support Your Strength

1. 'Even Breathing' or 'Box Breathing' to Steady Your Body, Mind and Emotions

Explore both of these to find out which works for you. You might find holding breath, as in box breathing, really energising and refreshing; some prefer not to hold their breath, in which case the 'even breathing' is better.

A. **Even breathing:** Breathe in and out to a slow count of 5 each way. Taking charge of your breathing can help you take charge of your mind, too, which can feel empowering. Give this a try for a minute or two to explore how it might work for you.

B. **Box breathing:** Breathe in for a slow count of 4, hold your breath for 4, then breathe out for 4 and hold for 4. Repeat 3–6 times. If you keep your chest slightly raised and hold your head up high while you breathe you can further boost your sense of strength and confidence. When you hold your breath, you trigger what is known as the 'diving reflex': your heart rate slows down and oxygen is shuttled to your vital organs to maintain their function. For short periods of time, such as a few seconds or minutes, this can feel energising. But, for maximum benefit, don't overdo holding your breath for more than you can comfortably manage.

2. Turn Around a Stress Response in a Matter of a Minute or So

A. Use deep, diaphragmatic breathing, which is the kind that makes your belly rise and your chest expand with each inhalation, followed by your chest and belly emptying with each exhalation. Enhance the breathing by pressing your belly in towards your spine to expel the last bit of air. Repeat a few times until you feel more in control, grounded and stronger in yourselb.

B. For a more powerful stress-relieving effect, you can more forcefully blow out your exhalation to release the build up of urgent energy. Focusing on exhalation and lengthening the outbreath will calm you down. It slows your heart rate and can settle restless or activated energy. This is because exhalation stimulates your parasympathetic 'rest and restore' branch of the nervous system that not only lowers heart rate but also lowers blood pressure and stress hormone levels in a matter of just a minute or twc.

C. Add an intention to release any negative feelings. With each long exhalation, send your worries out with your breath and clear your mind to think more clearly and resourcefully. Repeat a few times and then ask yourself how you would like to address the challenge that you facd.

D. Consciously releasing tension in your body while breathing can enhance the stress-relieving effect. When you catch yourself tensing up – such as in your jaw, shoulders, chest, belly – hold your breath to trigger your body to breathe again, and add some movement: gentle stretches or shaking out of tight areas to encourage your body to let go.

3. Dragon Breathing to Psych Yourself Up or to Release Anger

Breathe in through your nose and forcefully blow out each exhalation through your mouth. This practice can release tension and supercharge your energy. Speed up your breathing as fast as you like to psych yourself up and build courage to some challenge. Or you can slow your breathing down, especially if you want to control your anger. Continue for as long as it takes to release angry energy so that you can respond in an empowered, mature way.

4. From Sighs of Frustration to Exhales of Calm and Soothing

If you find yourself sighing in frustration or exasperation when someone or some situation really pushes your buttons, from shopping lines to insulting relatives, realise that these sighs are actually your autonomic nervous system trying to release tension and calm you down.

Knowing this can change how you react to the situation. Is it really worth all the tension it is causing in you? Or can you allow your body to at least stay energised and oxygenated and your mind clear through the frustrating moment for your own sake if nothing else? To emphasise the value of your sighs, take long, deep breaths, amplifying the sighs on exhalation as you visualise your frustration leaving you while peaceful calm and mental resilience grow in its place. Allow yourself a few good sighs to reset your nervous system back into balance. Feel free to include your voice to make your sigh feel as satisfying as possible. When you are around others this can be awkward, so either educate others about the value of sighing or carry this practice out in private.

5. From Self-doubt or Low Self-esteem to Feeling More Substantial

One breathing practice that can help here is full-body breathing. Self-doubt and low self-esteem live in our thoughts about ourselves and can cause us to shrink in our bodies. In this full-body breathing practice you are invited to imagine your natural breathing gradually spreading to permeate your entire body. Breathing in, you might imagine your whole body filling slightly from head to toe. Breathing out you might imagine your whole body emptying. If you are upright, retain a comfortable posture throughout. You can also use this breathing practice lying down, as a way to encourage more of your body to let go of tension and open to fuller breathing. Lying down, you can extend this breathing practice for 5–10 minutes for greater benefit. This exercise invites you to experience your three-dimensionality and the potential joy of vitality, rather than a two-dimensional image of yourself. The latter can fuel self-doubt and low self-esteem. Experiencing a three-dimensional version of self can promote appreciation of our bodies for how they carry us through life and help us achieve all we want from day to day.

6. Turn Anxiety Into Courage by Connecting With Breathing

Anxiety is perpetuated by worrisome thinking, so the simple act of turning attention away from thinking and into our bodies can be helpful. Breathing offers us one anchor. When we are anxious we hold our breath, which can build tension in our upper bodies. It can be helpful to imagine breathing into the lower belly and legs and even visualising each outbreath releasing all the way down into the ground through our legs and feet. Bending your knees slightly can help, or even bouncing slightly into your knees. You can also place both hands below your navel to help focus your awareness there. This practice can help to steady your mind, increase your grounding, grow your courage and ready you to perform better in what you need to. To add to your courage, raise your chest and hold your head up high. This posture tricks your brain into believing that you are strong and confident.

Supporting Vocal Strength

All the exercises in this chapter on centring, personal bubble or boundary, breathing and vocal strength all support each other. Here are some ideas focusing specifically on vocal strength.

Drop Your Weight Into Gravity and Speak With Greater Authority

Sit upright. Keep your spine straight and drop your centre of gravity down towards the ground so that you feel your weight sitting more heavily in your seat. Notice how you can speak with greater authority as your voice resonates from deeper inside your core.

To Support Public Speaking

When you speak, imagine projecting your voice outwards to fill the space around, which does not mean speaking loudly or shouting. (For public speaking you probably will have a microphone anyway.) You can play with this feeling in your spare time, too: speaking softly to engage with those close to you and throwing your voice out further to speak to people around a dinner table and further to a group you might be presenting to. You might experience how projecting your voice outwards, carried on a good deep exhalation and with your voice resonating from deep inside your belly, can boost your sense of confidence.

Power Up Your Voice With Good, Deep Breathing

Take a deep breath in and then send your message out clearly on a long exhalation. You can practise this in your spare time by singing your favourite song or humming your favourite tune. If you feel the emotion behind the tune, it can have the added benefit of helping you link to your emotions, to encourage speaking from your heart. This can have added impact to help convey our messages sincerely in any context.

Boost Sincerity in Your Speech

Along with being in touch with the emotions behind what you say, you can also boost sincerity at relevant times by placing a hand over your chest or heart area. Not only does this gesture convey sincerity it also encourages letting go of tension in the chest, throat and jaw, which can free up your ability to express yourself verbally.

Speak With Your Whole Body

Use arm gestures and shifts in posture to help emphasise your point while speaking. Explore the difference between full-body speaking and frozen-to-the-spot speaking, to experience the benefits of mobilising your body to help project your message.

Voice Warm-up Practice for Public Speaking

A practice that can help warm up your voice for clearer, more confident communication, such as for public speaking or presenting, is to articulate the vowel sounds. The following order takes into account *where* in the body the different sounds resonate, as a way to exercise your vocal cords with different kinds of sounds that you might use naturally in speech. Feel free to make up a spontaneous tune as you go along.

- ❁ **'I':** Repeat an 'I' sound a few times (as in referring to yourself as 'I') and feel how this sound can resonate up in the crown of your head.
- ❁ **'E':** Repeat an 'E' sound as in the word 'eel' and you can also play with it as an 'E' sound as in the word 'egg'. Repeat a few times and notice how this sound seems to concentrate and resonate in your throat area.
- ❁ **'A':** Repeat an 'A' sound, as in 'aaah', opening your mouth to project your voice and feeling how this letter can open and resonate in your chest area.
- ❁ **'O':** Repeat an 'O' sound as in the word 'open' and feel how this sound can resonate in your belly area.
- ❁ **'U':** Repeat a 'U' sound as in the word 'you' and feel how this sound can resonate down in your pelvic bowl.

Feel free to play with these sounds in any way that you like, perhaps alternating moving from 'I' to 'U' and then in reversing from 'U' to 'I' a few times, or mixing up the sounds spontaneously.

One more classic voice practice from yoga is the Aum or Om sound. This sound can centre us, relieve stress and bring a greater sense of inner peace. Take a deep breath in and slowly sound the Aum, ending with a long 'mmmmm' noticing the resonance of the sounds in your body as you move from 'Aaaauuuu' to 'mmmmm'. Repeat 3 times, making your Aum sound as long as you can on exhalation. Then, to maximise the experience, sit quietly for a few moments with eyes closed if you can and notice your body sensations.

CHAPTER 8

BOOSTING CREATIVITY AND ZEST FOR LIFE

'Creativity is intelligence having fun.'
ALBERT EINSTEIN

Creativity fosters our ability to see the world in novel ways, to think new thoughts, make new associations, perhaps discover hidden patterns or make new connections between things.

Creativity is something that we all possess and can draw on in our daily lives. It could involve coming up with ideas for dinner, choosing our clothes each day and adding creative touches to our home or website or birthday card. Or it could involve bigger creative endeavours like an artwork, writing a book, designing a scientific experiment or using creative visualisation to assist with new business ideas.

Creative expression tends to increase confidence and happiness, enhance our problem-solving ability, reduce stress and improve emotional resilience, mood and our sense of pride and self-esteem. Creative activities might also require us to slow down, offering welcome relief from a fast-paced life. At work, creativity can foster out-of-the-box thinking, improved problem-solving abilities and being more flexible and adaptable to change.

From a bio-chemical perspective, higher dopamine levels can drive our motivation and enthusiasm to explore our interests and to take interest in novel experiences. This is fuel for creativity. Highly creative people tend to have naturally higher dopamine levels. For those of us who are not highly creative naturally, however, dopamine levels can be increased through exposure to novelty and when we move towards things that feel exciting.

Creative thinking, especially 'aha' moments, spark activity in multiple brain areas at once. This has been referred to as our 'high-creative' network. It is seen to include: our default brain network, engaged when we allow our mind to wander or daydream; our executive network stimulated when we focus or control our thought processes; and our salience network, which helps us switch between our default and executive networks while immersed in creative thinking. This is different from non-creative times when the activation of one network causes the deactivation of others. For example, when we focus on work admin our executive network is active but our default, daydreaming network is deactivated and vice versa.

With practice we all can improve on our ability to be creative, for example by including daily opportunities for creative thinking, brainstorming or artistic expression.

5 Ways Physical Movement Boosts Creativity and Zest for Life

There is another way that we can stimulate creative thinking and that is through physical movement. Our bodies play an important role in keeping our creative juices and zest for life flowing. Following are some examples that you might experiment with to help you tap into your creativity.

1. Go for a Walk or Have a Walking Meeting

Both the founder of Apple, the late Steve Jobs and Facebook's Mark Zuckerberg were/are known for making use of walking meetings to inspire ideas. A Stanford study showed that the generation of creative ideas is significantly boosted while walking and for a short period after. The walking-creativity link has been associated with divergent thinking, which is the art of generating many ideas as possibilities, compared with convergent thinking, which is the art of evaluating, analysing, organising and selecting from the ideas we come up with. So next time your creativity needs a boost, try taking a break, going for a walk and applying your mind to what feels most important. On the flip side, studies have noted that walking is not good for our ability to focus (which draws on convergent rather than divergent thinking and benefits more from our holding still and focusing). So go for a walk when you want to get ideas flowing and then sit down and be still to focus your mind to choose from, evaluate or develop the ideas that you have come up with.

2. Loosen Up or Shake Out Your Body

In the same way that walking stimulates creative, divergent thinking, any kind of fluid movement can do the same. A study carried out in 2012 by Michael L. Slepian and Nalini Ambady found that fluid arm movement led to enhanced creative generation, remote association and cognitive flexibility. It also can have an energising effect on us. As a quick way to boost your energy levels and spark some of dopamine's zest for life, such as during a focused day at work, you might pause now and again to loosen up or shake out your body. This can have a refreshing effect on mind and body.

3. Talk With Your Hands

Another way to focus on physical movement in service of creativity and clear communication is through hand movements. Hand movements are found to stimulate creative and more productive thinking than when we hold our hands still while speaking. This is something you might try next time you brainstorm ideas on your own or talk things through with a friend or colleague. Include your hands and compare this with holding your hands still. Which promotes a better flow of thoughts?

4. Lean Forwards

When we physically lean even slightly forwards it tends to focus our minds on the future, as opposed to when we lean backwards, according to research by Lynden K. Miles, Louise K. Nind and C. Neil Macrae in 2010. This study, related to the field of embodied cognition, explored how our metaphors tend to arise from our physical experience. Exploring phrases such as *'You have your whole future ahead of you'* and *'Keep moving forward and leave the past behind you'* showed that people tend to lean slightly forwards when thinking of the future and slightly backwards when thinking about the past, as if the past and future were physically in front or behind us. So if you're feeling down or stuck, you might use this knowledge to your advantage by leaning forwards and inviting your mind to focus on helpful plans and ideas for your future.

5. Jump for Joy!

This is one of the best ways for you to boost happiness and fire up feelings of excitement. In turn this positivity can open your mind to creativity. Creative regular opportunities for improving agility and buoyancy in the way that jumping or rebounding in any way facilitates can improve our resilience for bouncing back from setbacks and it can add a spring to our step. We might jump for joy or jump on a trampoline. We might also cultivate our springiness while we jog or with a skipping rope, or in an exercise class, or on the sports field, or on a dance floor, or simply bopping to the beat. Any opportunity can do the trick. It has also been shown that imagining jumping can lift our mood in the same way as actually jumping. This offers a great way to shift our mood even when we are not able to move much, such as when sitting in a car or at the office. Simply imagine happiness and your mood will follow.

Client Story

Boosting Creativity and Dissolving Frustration by Freeing Up the Body

Janice is the director of a small business. At one point in our coaching work we applied dopamine-stimulating skills that included loosening up her body to help her work more productively and creatively with a member of her team. This team member, who we'll call Faye, was invaluable to the business and she really triggered Janice.

At the start of this piece of work, Janice was feeling irritable and frustrated. She described how Faye was the main reason for this. Janice found Faye to be irresponsible, testy and regularly undermining of her authority. This was suspected as linked with Faye having been in the business for longer than Janice. As Janice spoke, practically through gritted teeth, her body looked as tense as she felt stuck about what to do.

On paying attention to her body language at my invitation, she quickly picked up on her high levels of tension. I asked her to contrast her tense posture by shaking out and loosening up her body to explore how this physical shift could impact on her state of mind. Janice shook and stretched out her body for a few moments and then slumped back in her seat – something I had never seen her do to this extent. She described how freeing it felt. It even made her laugh at the possibility of loosening and lightening up in this physical way. Knowing that physical movement can free up creative thinking, I immediately took the opportunity to ask her to brainstorm ways she might respond differently to Faye, asking her to come up with a few different ideas even if they felt crazy. Janice started by poking some fun at the thought of telling Faye off and firing her, although she immediately over-ruled this thought because of how valuable Faye was to the business. Her second thought was how freeing it could feel if she literally sat back more in meetings where Faye was present, to help her avoid responding to every irritation. This inspired her to breathe more fully and her eyes lit up with the idea. I encouraged her to continue thinking creatively and after a few moments another idea sprang to mind about coming up with a longer-term vision in which they did not need to work so closely together in the business. Janice shared how she had been hired to turn the business around by putting structures and processes in place for the long-term sustainability of the business. This was a role that would change once these goals were met probably within a couple of years. Then Janice might move on to a different area of the business or perhaps another business opportunity entirely in which she could apply her particular skillset. As she spoke, she realised how difficult Faye must find all the changes. This stirred up compassion as Janice realised how much freedom and authority Faye had enjoyed in the business previously. Janice spontaneously took a deep breath and in that moment her motivation increased to remain patient with Faye. In the meantime she also realised that she had allies on her team. These were other managers who she could draw on to help her communicate with Faye. This would reduce their contact hours as another way to help with what might simply be a personality clash between them.

Following our brainstorming, Janice decided, for a start, to try out her idea of sitting back more than usual in her next team meeting. On reporting back to me after the meeting she said it was far less stressful than usual. The laid-back posture had helped her to realise that she did not need to jump in so quickly with responses. This also allowed her to speak from a place of quiet authority when she did speak as opposed to high irritation. It felt as if a huge load had been lifted off her shoulders as she discovered her ability to resist getting hooked by every seemingly silly question or provocation. This tied in with an area for growth in her leadership, to work on relationship building, which tended to be limited by her irritability and impatience.

As Janice explored releasing tension and relaxing her posture, such as by pausing to loosen up her body now and again through the work day, it seemed to naturally help her feel lighter and happier, often placing a smile on her face too. Over time this intervention led Janice to realise that her quick, intelligent mind could benefit from time for creative reflection to spark different ideas and approaches to situations. It also helped to curtail her belief in 'My way or the highway.' This not only reduced her own stress levels, it also led to feedback from others that she had become more approachable and less intimidating. As for her relationship with Faye, they might never work easily together, but the volatility of their interactions settled and they even found their way to a heartfelt conversation soon after our coaching sessions on this topic. Janice initiated the conversation out of her newly found compassion and it seemed that Faye really appreciated the opportunity to be heard around how hard she was finding all the changes. Janice shared how having this conversation changed the mood between them for the better.

The Creative Benefits of Coming to Your Senses

'Your senses are a doorway to the present moment Instead of defaulting to browsing your phone, open your five senses. Feel the air on your skin. Smell nature's scents. See the beauty in the leaves. Breathe in and taste the air. Touch your soft skin. Connect to now.'

MELISSA MONTE

This mindful technique may not use physical movement, but it does invite us to come into our bodies and experience the world more through our senses, such as through sight, sound, smell and touch. This is as opposed to getting lost in our thoughts about our experience. 'Coming to our senses' is another way to open up creativity and divergent thinking networks in our brains.

Here is one of my examples. One morning I set out for a walk with the intention of getting some exercise and fresh air. The wind was chilly and I instinctively slipped my hands into my pockets. I was halfway around the park before I realised that I had been lost in thought. Decisions were made, children were considered and inspiration flickered with new ideas for work. I noticed a slight headache beginning behind my eyes and that my shoulders were raised as my arms pulled tightly in at my sides to fend off the cold.

I remembered the value of pausing to take in my surroundings, through my senses. What were the sights around me? I looked around, noticing trees and fresh green grass and a bird flying in the sky. I noticed houses and cars across the road, and in the large park there were a few dogs running free, chasing balls or each other with their owners nearby. What were the sounds? I listened near and far to birds chirping, traffic whizzing by, a car horn suddenly startling me, and the faint rustling of leaves in the trees. I was aware of the sense of touch of cold air. I also could feel my heartbeat pumping warmth and energy through me, from the physical exertion of my walk. I spontaneously took my hands out my pockets. My shoulders and neck relaxed as my arms began to swing at my sides. I also considered what smells and tastes were with me at the time.

Our five senses give us information in different ways. There is never a dull moment when we tune into this sensory level of our experience. There are always so many sensory opportunities available to us from our environment and from inside our body and mind. There is also a sixth sense that can be experienced as a heart or gut sense of what is going on around us. This is a level of our experience that might be hard to explain, yet it is available to us all. It informs how safe we feel in the moment, nudging us to move towards what we feel curious about and away from what we feel threatened by.

As I became more aware of my different senses, in the moment, I began to feel a tingle of vitality rising inside me. Focused, head-down determination when I was lost thought had turned to a new spring in my step. My body felt more open and upright and my movement more fluid. My breathing felt energised and my mind was clear. The dull headache from the start of my walk had dissolved.

I invited my mind to return to the thoughts that were with me at the start of my walk so that I could reconsider them from my new broader perspective. I considered how I might see my situation differently, who I might be able to speak with for helpful input, what possible options there might be for solving my challenges and what my gut or heart were communicating with me about my situation. As I considered my options, my mind fanned out to explore new possibilities. My mind and body also felt more expansive and relaxed as helpful solutions came to light. Even just this was relieving.

Coming to Your Senses for a New Perspective

To come to your senses and explore what doing this might have to offer you, you are invited to pause for a moment to look around and notice your surroundings through fresh eyes. Reach out to touch one or two things around you to wake up your sense of touch. Listen to the sounds around you. Notice the taste in your mouth and the smell in the air. Notice sensations in your body and perhaps the temperature of the air or the feeling of the clothes on your skin or the comfort of your posture. How do you feel now that you are more present through your senses? If you have been distracted or struggling through some work or a home situation, how might your new sensory clarity help you address things differently? You can also include your heart and gut in assessing your situation to add more potentially useful insights.

*Helpful Workout Recommendation
(In the workout section at the end of this book)

WORKOUT FOR BOOSTING CREATIVE ENERGY
AGILITY WORKOUT OPTIONS FOR ADDING A SPRING TO YOUR STEP

CHAPTER 9

KEEPING ENERGY AND MOTIVATION FLOWING

*'Keep your eyes on the stars, and
your feet on the ground.'*

THEODORE ROOSEVELT

This chapter hones in on the art of creating a steady flow of dopamine to energise us to achieve our goals. It draws on dopamine's role both as a motivation and reward molecule. The practices of this chapter can enhance our go-getter spirit by inviting us to dream up exciting, inspiring goals and regularly top up on our excitement, energy and motivation as we move towards our goals. The practices are divided into four key areas:

1. **Dreaming:** Coming up with exciting ideas that you can translate into goals to strive towards.
2. **Persevering:** Keeping up energy, motivation and regular actions towards achieving your goals.
3. **Exploring:** Drawing on fresh and new ways of experiencing the moment to stimulate dopamine's motivation and curiosity.

4. **Celebrating:** Rewarding and celebrating your achievements of long and short-term goals, as well as small wins along the way.

These categories do tend to overlap and cycle back on each other as we move through life, working together to keep our spirits lifted and our energy refreshed at different times and in different situations.

1. Dreaming: Practices to Support Dreaming Up Exciting Ideas

All of our exciting aspirations start from a dream or a vision that we hold in our minds. This vision is what stimulates dopamine and magnetises us to move towards it, especially when it feels truly exciting or inspiring. To get dopamine flowing in this way, you can reflect on what excites you or aligns with your values or what you feel really passionately about. This could involve dreaming big, such as tuning into your core purpose in life and how you might apply your unique talents. Dreaming big in this way can really boost a sense of life well lived. Tuning in to what excites you in the shorter term is also key to be able to regularly uplift your spirits and perhaps put a spring in your step. This could be anything, such as planning and looking forward to a well-deserved holiday, or quality time to spend with loved ones who you might not get to see so often or even shorter term planning for fun and meaningful entertainment on the weekend. It could also be getting excited about something that you would really like to buy and working towards getting it. So long as it puts a twinkle in your eyes and has a motivating and energising effect, it can do the trick of keeping dopamine flowing.

In relation to dopamine's excitement and motivation to achieve some reward, it's important to remember that dopamine works best in happy balance with other bio-chemicals. To avoid burn-out or addictive behaviour it is important to listen to your body and your energy levels and allow time for serotonin-stimulating rest, recuperation and integration, for testosterone's strength building for a boost to courage, focus and stamina along the way, as well as allowing time for oxytocin's nurturing and leaning into support systems along the way.

A Visualisation Process

It is recommended to read through this visualisation to stir your mind into how you might respond. Then when you have time, set aside half an hour or longer for big life topics, to allow you to delve into that area of your life through this visualisation. Of course you are welcome to return to the process as many times as necessary to fuel dopamine's fire, such as when life might veer into feeling boring or stagnant or to continue to develop on a visualisation that you have already started.

What might you visualise today?

- Your core purpose or deeper sense of meaning, such as how to use your skills and talents to the best of your ability at this time in a way that feels personally meaningful.
- Something to look forward to, to uplift your spirits, such as planning a well-deserved holiday or quality time with important people who you might not get to see so often.
- Some big change, such as a new work opportunity or the experience of living in another country or embarking on a new study and career path.
- Or it could be coming up with ideas for rewarding yourself for your perseverance or achievement in the above, such as by planning to purchase something meaningful or arrange for an enjoyable experience, such as a night out at the theatre or a massage or attending a workshop for personal growth.

Once you have chosen something to focus on, ask yourself how you might go about achieving it to activate your initial ideas. Then loosen up your body and free up tension to stimulate your creative mind (as suggested in the previous chapter) for going deeper into your creative visualisation. Here are a few ideas to guide you:

- As you follow the paths of your creative thinking and planning, allow your visualisations to feel alive in your mind's eye, like a dream that you can follow with curiosity and excitement. This can feel really energising, adding to your dopamine boost.
- You can enhance your visualisation and encourage yourself to stay a little longer with it for more of a dopamine boost, by adding visual detail like colour and environment: who is with you, your circumstance, your home, your work surrounds or whatever feels relevant. The more you infuse your imagination with dream-like elements that are attractive to you, the more your dopamine drive can wake up to entice you to move towards your goal.
- You can further develop your imaginative process by calling on any of your five senses: sight, sound, smell, taste and how you feel in your dream circumstance (touch). Include as much sensory detail as possible, as if you are really there.

❊ When you arrive at your goals in real life, the dream sparkle can sometimes wear off and reality can set in with all its challenges and rewards. The same can apply when you might not achieve your goals, which might need re-evaluation or re-visioning. If this happens, take some time to reconnect with your visualisation process and with the next inspiring dream in order to step back onto the dopamine treadmill.

❊ To embody your visualisation and anchor it more strongly in your physical experience, pause at the end of your inspiring visualisation and notice where in your body you can sense feeling. This awareness can become a cue to reconnect you back to your goals. To find a physical cue you can either place your hand on your body where your positive, inspiring feelings feel strongest or you can use a hand gesture or body posture that can be reused at any time in the days to come as a quick reminder of your inspiring vision and to give your dopamine another quick boost.

For the longer-term goals that relate to, for example, life purpose or meaningful work change, you could repeat these visualisation suggestions in relation to the longer and shorter term. For example you might visualise yourself 10 years from now and then repeat the visualisation as 5 years from now and then 2 years and then what the present or very short term can look like if you were to include elements or actions in your life that align with your longer-term goals.

2. Persevering: Practices to Support Perseverance Towards Meaningful Goals

Following are some tips that can help you persevere towards meaningful dreams and goals. They can help you to keep up your energy and motivation, building excitement and 'pinging' your brain's reward system as regularly as you need.

Visualise Success

This technique is popular with many sports people, theatre performers, public speakers and actors. It involves picturing or simulating in your mind, in great detail, the successful outcome, such as of a performance, including the masterful execution of all the actions and words involved and soaking up the experience of the great applause or praise at the end. The more we can embody these feelings, the more we can unstick old, limiting patterns and replace them with new and helpful ones. Then you can arrive at the time of actually performing or presenting feeling like you've done it many times before. Let's take the example of public speaking: you might picture what you are wearing and how you stand, waiting to come on stage or in front of your audience. Then you picture how you stride out in front of your audience and enter into your presentation, from greeting to closing, and even picturing how the audience responds, allowing your body to take it all in. This part can be tricky if you are in the habit of imagining your smallness or limitations. It might take some practise to open to a mindset of success.

We can use this visualisation as regularly as feels helpful. It draws on the power of our imagination to stimulate the same neural networks as performing in real life.

It should be noted, however, our drive to succeed is just one aspect of a multi-faceted life. If our sense of worth is only measured by professional success, for example, then the ups and downs natural to any profession will cut into us more deeply. Self-worth is far more stable when it is grounded in our core identity, or spirituality or family values. According to seasoned businessman Ben Sigelman this perspective can actually be good for business. In his words: 'Make sure the core of your identity and your sense of self-worth is tied to something more grounded than your company's valuation. Ironically, that's the best way to set yourself up for the risk-taking you'll need to maximise it.'

Ensure Pleasure Beats Willpower

How you view the hard work that goes into achieving your goals can make all the difference. It's natural to seek out and move towards pleasure and try to avoid pain. But if you can turn drudgery into exciting challenge, you can keep dopamine flowing. There are many creative ways to facilitate this transformation. You can make use of incentives or rewards to give you something tangible to work towards. This could be personal such as looking forward to a soak in the bath with bath salts at the end of a challenging day or booking a massage after a stressful week or planning to eat out at your favourite restaurant if you meet your target. Or it could be a shared reward such as financial incentives in the workplace to reach certain targets.

Another way to maintain enthusiasm or have your load feel lighter is by inserting mini-moments for enjoyable activities through your days. Always waiting for the perfect time to relax and enjoy yourself might not be as effective as building a sense of regular enjoyment and fun. For example, you might add to the enjoyment of a break from work by going for a longer-than-usual walk or calling a friend for a quick chat or listening to an inspiring podcast. Or you might increase your sense of enjoyment of your day by getting up a bit earlier to exercise in your favourite way and/or meditate so that you increase your sense of feeling fresh and ready for the day. In these kinds of ways you can regularly 'ping' your brain's reward and motivation system. Not only can this increase your enjoyment of life, it can also boost your stress resilience because of the rise in dopamine's energy, creativity and enthusiasm to help you through.

Complete Daily To-do Lists

You can also boost dopamine when you complete daily chores like cleaning your kitchen after meals or getting through the laundry or spring-cleaning a part of your house. Or in the workplace it could be getting through what you want to accomplish in the day. Any time you have a sense of completion, no matter how small or tedious, it can give you a hit of dopamine satisfaction that can motivate you to continue being productive.

Set Regular, Time-bound Deadlines

Feeling the rush of deadlines approaching is a dopamine-boosting experience. This does not mean we should make a habit of leaving everything to the last minute; rather, it means that rising to a challenge can feel exciting. When we break down long-term goals into short-term achievable steps and set a timeline that we can tick items off of along the way, it can help with perseverance towards our long-term goals by keeping our dopamine and motivation levels regularly topped up by our short-term achievements. Another way to increase your motivation and accountability is to let someone else know about your goals. This could be someone in your personal life or in a professional context. In some work contexts this is incorporated into regular business practice as work goals become key performance indicators, linked with performance appraisals and tied to incentives that all feed into employee accountability and motivation.

3. Exploring: Practices to Stimulate Dopamine in Daily Life

When you experience something as if for the first time it can open up what Buddhists refer to as *beginner's mind*, which is an attitude of perhaps child-like curiosity and motivation to explore life, new places and new situations without preconceived ideas. This is another simple way to stimulate dopamine that also can come about naturally when we live in a more present and mindful way. To get a sense of this, you might think of driving the streets of your hometown and how time can easily pass with you lost in thought and barely noticing your surroundings. Compare this with walking the streets of a place you have never been to, perhaps a holiday destination, and the attention to detail and quality of presence that you bring to this novel situation. This curiosity to explore can feel rewarding in itself and it can be motivating too. Here are a few ideas for stimulating beginner's mind in daily life:

- If you like to exercise outdoors, such as running, walking or cycling, choose new routes now and again.
- Explore different parts of your hometown or go on road trips or holidays that inspire you to discover new things.
- Wherever you are, open your senses and be really present to your environment to take in your environment and your experience more fully.
- Take up a new hobby.
- Explore the creative arts. If you find a modality that you particularly enjoy, use it regularly.
- Play! Games of any kind can feel new and fun each time you play them.
- Follow a recipe for a new meal one night a week.
- Try something you've never tried before!

4. Celebrating: Celebrating Achievements Big and Small

Following are some tips for celebrating your achievements, big and small, to maximise the dopamine experience.

Celebrate Big Achievements

Celebrating reaching big goals is important. How we each choose to acknowledge our victories can differ. You could celebrate with others or gift yourself with something you have been wanting for a long time. Any way that you allow yourself to bask in a sense of achievement can be a great stimulant for dopamine and motivation to achieve again in future.

Celebrate Smaller Wins Along the Way

Celebrating your smaller wins along the way with short- and medium-term goals is also a great way to keep dopamine and motivation flowing. This can be helped by breaking work goals up into weekly and daily to-do lists (then as suggested above you get your dopamine boost from completing your to-do list). You could also reward your small wins with enjoyable experiences such as suggested earlier in the point about pleasure beating willpower and incentivising yourself with something to look forward to.

Raise Your Arms in Victory

Each time you reach a small or large goal you can amplify your dopamine experience by physically expressing the 'Yes, I did it!' feeling. You can do so in any way that feels good, such as holding a fist and bringing your elbow in to your side with your 'Yes!' or by raising your arms in a victory pose, as an athlete would spontaneously do on a victory lap after a big win. This can be an action just a few seconds long to help your brain register and amplify your sense of achievement. Because of the power of imagination to stimulate the same neural pathways as real actions, you could also just imagine doing so for your dopamine boost, such as when your situation does not allow for an excited victory lap! Next time you have a sense of achievement give this a try, holding your arms up high and inviting yourself to open more fully to dopamine's exhilaration.

*Helpful Workout Recommendation
(In the workout section at the end of this book)

WORKOUT FOR STRENGTHENING YOUR REACH AND PERSEVERANCE

CHAPTER 10

WARMHEARTEDNESS FOR OURSELVES AND EACH OTHER

'The best and most beautiful things in the world cannot be seen or even touched – they must be felt with the heart.'

HELEN KELLER

This chapter is about nurturing a sense of loving interconnectedness through the oxytocin-stimulating warmth of our hearts. Warmth is both literal and metaphoric. When we literally feel warm, like when we soak in a warm bath or snuggle up under a warm blanket, feelings associated with oxytocin are found to increase such as trust, intimacy and loving-kindness. When we metaphorically feel warm or loving and compassionate towards ourselves and each other our body temperature can also rise.

The physiology of the heart can inspire another metaphoric lesson around the importance of balancing giving and receiving. The job of the heart is to sustain life. It does so by continuously pumping nutrient-rich blood and fresh oxygen from the lungs to nourish the body's tissues as well as removing waste products. The pathways for keeping this vital nourishment flowing not only serve the rest of the body, they also cycle back through the heart. This can apply to self-care too – by absorbing so that we can then extend outwards. The practices in this chapter cycle between self-care and extending our care towards others.

Take a moment to feel into this cycle of giving and receiving through your heart by imagining a favourite person or a pet in your life, or a cute baby or baby animal – something that melts your heart. Allow the warmth that this image generates to spread outwards and fill your whole body, possibly extending further to fill the space around you or even spreading far out into the world. Bask for a few moments in this warmth.

Effects of heart-based feelings on health and wellbeing

The HeartMath Institute is an organisation that researches the effects of heart-based feelings on health and wellbeing, relationships and influence on a global level. In one of their studies, a group of participants was taught a meditation practice and asked to connect their breathing and positive thoughts to the heart. Significant increases in DHEA, an anti-aging hormone, were measured, as well as a decrease in the stress hormone cortisol. Health improvements were also recorded in the participants with cardiac histories and symptoms of depression and anxiety.

Not only does feeling loving-kindness from our hearts affect us personally, it has also been shown to spread out to influence those around us. Looking into this, a group of researchers – Shaltout, Tooze, Rosenberger and Kemper – showed that the practice of loving-kindess meditation increased parasympathetic regulation (in other words had a calming effect) in both the meditator and the control group of participants who were in the same room but unaware of being sent thoughts of loving-kindness. So our individual practice has the potential to quietly and positively touch the lives of others.

The HeartMath Institute is a leader in taking this ripple effect of the heart to yet another level through their Global Coherence Initiative (GCI). The aim of the GCI is to shift global consciousness from discord and instability to balance, cooperation and enduring peace, through heart-focused and compassionate projects. They measure the heart's influence in electromagnetic terms and have found that the electromagnetic field emitted by the heart is stronger than from any other part of the body and many times stronger than the field emitted by the brain. The GCI seeks to focus and draw on the collective electromagnetic power of our hearts as a change agent in the world towards peace and harmony. The GCI also has a goal of furthering our understanding of the energetic interconnectedness between humanity, the Earth's magnetic field and other planetary energetic fields. In general, data from HeartMath Institute studies is yielding promising results. Personally, I find this an inspiring reminder to harness the power of my heart. Some days all I need is some heart for myself or for those close by. Other days my heart can open for all and our planet.

Short Practice

Breathing Through Your Heart and Directing Compassion Towards Yourself and Others

Inspired by a technique used by the HeartMath Institute, here is a breathing exercise that can be done any time and anywhere for an oxytocin boost through heart-centred breathing.

Sit in a comfortable position. Read through the instructions and then close your eyes (if you are comfortable to do so) to focus on the practice more deeply. If you have limited time and so that you can focus more deeply on the practice, set a timer to alert you when your time has run out, or continue for as long as you wish when you are able.

- Move your awareness into your heart. You might imagine taking an elevator from your head down to your heart.

- When you get there, pause to feel into being there as if you could look around inside the energy centre of your heart and orient yourself there.

- Turn your attention to your natural breathing and imagine that your breathing moves in and out through your heart centre. As you do so, encourage your chest to expand in all directions with each inhalation (front, back and sides) and relax with each exhalation.

- Add an image of someone you love or a place that easily warms your heart, and hold this in mind to amplify the heartwarming effect. If you struggle to come up with something, call to mind the cutest thing that you can think of, perhaps a newborn baby or a tiny puppy or kitten, and allow this to warm your heart.

- Breathing for coherence: While focusing on breathing through your heart centre, slow down your breathing to breathe in for a count of 5 and out for a count of 5. Research through the HeartMath Institute confirms that when you are feeling stressed, as little as 3–5 minutes of this kind of heart-focused breathing can effectively shift our heart rhythm into greater coherence, with many benefits: it is good for our physical health; we have better access to our higher intelligence so that we can see our situations more clearly and optimistically; and emotionally it is associated with feelings such as sincere appreciation, gratitude, compassion and love.

- Optional extra: If you have been going through a challenging time, after breathing through your heart for a few minutes as above you can imagine breathing your challenging situation through your heart to lend it some heartfelt compassion. This can also open up a new attitude and perhaps bring some new ideas, too, for how to address your situation.

For a boost to self-love and self-compassion: Shower your loving feelings into yourself, absorbing heartfelt warmth from head to toe as thoroughly as you can. Compassion has been defined by Pema Chödrön as the ability to be with pain, your own and that of others, with an open mind and an open heart. With this idea in mind, of an open heart even when in pain, you might take the time now and again through your days to send love especially to parts of yourself that hurt (physically or emotionally) or that are not so well. This kind of heartfelt support, with the feel-good bio-chemistry that it can generate, has been found beneficial, such as potentially supporting recovery, reducing pain, improving our attitude towards our circumstance and motivation to be proactive.

For a boost in compassion towards others: Hold specific people in mind and send loving feelings out towards them and you can send loving kindness out to communities or parts of the world or to the world as a whole, as a kind of heart-based subtle activism. Subtle activism is a term used to describe the application of spiritual or consciousness-based practices as a contribution towards collective transformation.

For a quick boost to self-empowerment when feeling overwhelmed or triggered: Take a moment, even while on the go, such as after reading or listening to troubling news or when seeing someone in need, to quietly send compassion or good wishes out to the person or situation. This can help you to feel stronger in a heartfelt way, as opposed to slipping into being emotionally triggered or overwhelmed.

To Be Compassionate or to Criticise? That is the Question

Some believe that being overly compassionate, accepting and kind towards ourselves will slow us down or reduce our motivation and drive to achieve our goals in life. Some believe that it will make us weak or encourage us to not take responsibility. Many think that being harsh on ourselves when we fail or make mistakes is the best way to pick ourselves up and move forward again. Research, such as that of Dr Kristin Neff, shows that this is not true. The more kind-hearted we are towards ourselves, especially with setbacks or personal challenges, the better we can access our brain's intelligence, optimise our health and ultimately feel happier and more stable.

Compassion, directed towards ourselves or others, is a strength, not a weakness. It is found to motivate us and help us take more responsibility. It can also help us bounce back after setbacks. When we are more compassionate towards ourselves it is also found to make us more giving towards others, promoting pro-social behaviour. It might take some practise, but with time a heart-led life can come to feel natural.

Client Story

Picking Up Warmheartedness

Miles is an ambitious and successful businessman in his late forties. A number of things led him to realise that he needed to make some changes. He barely slept because of staying up late working and then struggled to turn his busy mind off for sleep; his diet was poor because he mostly ate on the go; he had not exercised regularly for a long time; and his weight had increased over the last few years. As a result, various physical and health issues had emerged. Along with this he was having relationship troubles with his wife, who had accused him of being unavailable, impatient and quick tempered.

Miles sat in my consulting room describing all of this in a deep, clear voice. As he spoke he looked me squarely in the eyes and maintained strength and uprightness in his spine even while sitting back in the chair. He ended with, 'I can accomplish so much every day and be very successful in business, but in my personal life and in taking care of my own health I am not doing so well.' For the first time in the session, he averted his eyes.

As our work progressed, Miles came to see how his body felt stuck in a fight response, vigilant and on the go all the time and not breathing very deeply. This served him well in the business world, but acted like a shield that protected him from feeling vulnerable. Miles came from a family where his father was largely unavailable, immersed in his own work and with a quick temper that Miles had inherited. His mother, although affectionate and emotionally attuned at times, was inconsistent in being there for him as she was busy raising three children and was jumpy around her husband's temper. So Miles learned from an early age to become his own person and take care of himself emotionally as best as he could.

After reflecting on his background, there was a moment of pause in which Miles slipped into dreaminess and shared about an unexpectedly impactful recent experience. He was at a friend's house and watched as soothing eucalyptus balm was rubbed onto their sick toddler's chest. Miles shared how he wished he had been that child receiving the balm and how wonderful that might be. I took this as a clue for how to proceed towards softening Miles's chronic fight response. I invited him to pause and soothingly rub his own chest as if applying balm. He closed his eyes and willingly did so, which later progressed into a soothing stroking motion of his arms and, eventually, with my visualisation guidance, to imagining his mother and even his father holding their arms out to him in welcome and support. His eyes welled up even though he sat up tall and tried his best to fight back the tears. Even so, a softening had opened in him as he began to feel his age-old longing for love and nurturing.

Some time later Miles shared how he had incorporated the self-soothing actions of rubbing his chest or stroking his arms as reminders whenever he thought of it during the day, to be calmer. He spoke of how he was beginning to know himself differently, too, as a result, considering all sorts of new things such as how to take better care of his health, including investing in a personal trainer and being more mindful about his food choices.

With my encouragement, another change started unfolding in his relationship with his wife too. First in our conversations and then with his wife he became more skilled at recognising and acknowledging the anxiety, fear and vulnerability that lay beneath his anger. He came to see how underneath his strong and shielded exterior lived a scared, young part of himself that found comfort in the distraction of being busy and always on the move, which later in life translated into an ambitious drive to succeed. When he would acknowledge to his wife 'I am feeling anxious' rather than shouting at her, it generated a heartfelt softness in her towards him that usually led to a helpful discussion about the matter at hand as opposed to their history of spiraling into a fight.

Learning to manage his anxiety emerged as a clear theme for Miles's personal growth. A soothing hand to his heart gave him one quick remedy that he could use on his own. Added to this, his compassion grew towards his young self who seldom had anyone to reach out to. He knew that he did have someone to reach out to now – his wife, who loved him and wanted to reach out to him too, provided he softened enough to receive her. Together they felt inspired to develop their sense of mutual support in this new and tender way.

As with all personal change, the journey into tempering a very well-developed fight response and maintaining a more calm and heartfelt approach to life can be a lifelong process. Miles continues to slip up sometimes in his self-care and still remains a strong and driven businessman, but, for the most part, he is feeling enriched and happier in shifting towards a more heart-centred attitude to life.

*Helpful Workout Recommendation
(In the workout section at the end of this book)
HEART-OPENING WORKOUT

CHAPTER 11

10 WAYS TO BOOST OXYTOCIN AND WARMHEARTEDNESS

'When your heart opens the world around you changes.'

QIGONG MASTER MINGTONG GU

Whether you wish to counteract anxiety, prompt feeling more caring and nurturing towards yourself and others, or promote trust and cooperation, here are 10 proven ways to keep oxytocin flowing to support you.

1. Keep Warm

Enjoy a warm bath or shower before bed, bundle up in warm clothes if the weather is cold and snuggle with each other to share warmth. Any way you can keep warm and cosy can stimulate oxytocin.

2. Tell Dear People That You Love Them

Expressing our heart's feelings to significant others can give you an oxytocin boost.

3. Show That You Care

There are many ways to demonstrate affection and emotional support, from physical touch and hugs to giving gifts, helping another person and practising random acts of kindness. All have been associated with an increase in oxytocin levels in our bloodstreams.

4. Use Self-supportive Touch

Holding yourself or using touch in a nurturing way, such as placing a hand over your heart or holding your own hand when you feel nervous or massaging your temples when you are experiencing mental strain, can increase oxytocin levels as effectively as the touch of others. Or for emotional containment, you might try the 'over-under' self-hug, described in an earlier client story. This involves a self-hug in which your right hand is under your left armpit, palm against your rib cage, and your left hand is over your right upper arm. Touch works because your skin is like a superhighway to influencing your nervous system. In utero, your skin developed out of the same tissue as your nervous system, which is how the intimate relationship between skin and nervous system began. When carried out with care, touch can have a calming effect on us and increase our oxytocin levels in a matter of seconds, and if we can maintain our touch for 10 seconds or more it can be even more effective. It can be empowering to discover that there is something that you can do to help yourself, or at least until you can seek support from others.

5. Spend Time With Your Pet

For maximum oxytocin benefit, pat your dog or spend time physically holding your pet if possible. Engaging with your pet in loving, nurturing ways is a proven way to stimulate oxytocin. You can get an oxytocin boost from spending time with any animal even if not your own, so you might take any opportunity to say hello and pat or cuddle animals that you meet through your day. When we feel fondly towards animals, being in contact with them can quickly slow down our heart and breathing rates and lift our spirits in a way that is good for our health.

6. Keep a Gratitude Journal

Grow heart energy by focusing on that which you appreciate or are grateful for each day (such as writing three points at the end of each day that reflect on what was positive about the day). This practice can help you maintain a positive outlook and warm your heart on a regular basis.

7. Meditate With a Focus on Loving Kindness

More so than other forms of meditation, those that draw on extending your heart's warmth, kindness and compassion to others are most effective at stirring the heart and generating oxytocin. A Buddhist practice called tonglen, translated as loving-kindness meditation, is an example of a technique that has been studied extensively for its effectiveness, such as in promoting pro-social behaviour and emotional wellbeing as well as toning our nervous system in a way that supports sustainable happiness. The focus of this meditation is basically on sending out loving energy and good wishes towards others and into the world.

8. Have Some Face-to-face Time

When we spend time with people who we feel safe around and kindly towards it tends to boost our oxytocin levels. This in turn builds our sense of emotional connection. Meeting friends over coffee or going for a walk together can do the trick, as well as eating meals together and taking the time to ask about each other's days.

9. Lend Your Support Where You Can

This can be a challenging way that oxytocin is stimulated as it draws on the suffering of others and high-stress situations. Shared stressful or traumatic experiences like natural disasters raise oxytocin levels because they tend to pull people together, such as uniting survivors to support each other and attracting support from far and wide. This is probably a survival instinct based on strength in numbers and the survival value of reaching out to others for support. It has also been found that strong social support for victims directly following traumatic experience can prevent PTSD from setting in. This can be an invitation to all of us to lend a hand where we can and show that we care, especially when others are going through a tough time. It can be both for their benefit and our own.

10. Build Rapport Whenever You Can

Rapport is the feeling of positive emotional connection between people. Oxytocin loves heartfelt connection, so any opportunity to connect warmly and create rapport with others can be for our mutual benefit. Rapport can sometimes flow naturally and sometimes you might need to work at the connection. Here are a few physical skills to support the non-verbal side of rapport:

- **Give undivided attention** when in conversation as well as in greeting. Make an effort to focus all of your attention on the person you are with. It can feel so rewarding to the receiver of this attention and can win you favour towards good rapport going forwards.
- **Convey kindness** through your eyes and even a small smile on your face. This can be picked up on from a distance, so walk into a room prepared.
- **Listen with your heart** for emotional undertones to a person's words that you might respond to when appropriate, such as with a question like 'Are you ok?' or 'Is there anything I can do to help?' if someone clearly is upset. Mirroring a person's body language is one way to help you listen into and gain a felt sense of the emotional world of the person you are with. Just for a few moments, take on their posture. This can also convey emotional resonance in a primal and non-verbal kind of way, causing the person you are with to feel seen and understood, which is an ingredient for rapport. As an example of how this supports rapport, if you watch friends rapt in conversation you can easily notice from their degree of physical matching if they are in rapport or not. With mirroring, however, be careful not to stick with the other person's posture for too long or else you might come across as inauthentic.
- **Expand your ability to build rapport, especially if you hold a leadership role.** This involves, over time, developing your ability to be grounded, strong, fluid and expressive, and warm so as to be able to connect with people of different personality types that tend to match these various qualities. In this way, even though you have your own personality and do want to play to your strengths, you will find it easier to adapt your communication style when you need to, in order to build rapport and win favour with more people whom you lead.

CHAPTER 12

BOUNCING BACK FROM STRESS AND TONING YOUR NERVOUS SYSTEM FOR HAPPINESS

'The great thing, then, in all education, is to make our nervous system our ally instead of our enemy.'

WILLIAM JAMES

Life is not about eliminating stress. Stress is often what propels us to achievement and growth. What we want is to be able to notice more quickly when we are triggered and then choose to put our best foot forward to respond to our situation. We are hardwired to have our instinctual body take the lead quickly in emergency situations. But because of the high stress and intensity that modern life can bring, there may be times when every day can feel like an emergency situation. Our stress responses like fight or flight can be triggered regularly, which is exhausting – physically and emotionally.

From a bio-chemical point of view this kind of stress is taxing on your adrenal glands, which produce adrenaline to prepare your body for fight or flight. Adrenaline gives an initial surge of energy when you are triggered. Then cortisol levels quickly increase to help you rise to the challenge of stress and persevere towards safety. If stress were fleeting, your body would regain balance fairly quickly and easily after the threat has passed. But if stress is prolonged or perpetuated daily, it can throw your cortisol system chronically out of balance.

We are not designed to live in stress and survival mode for more than about half an hour at a time. Sure, it can feel exhilarating for a while, which is why some love the thrill of activities like bungee jumping and riding rollercoasters, but the adrenaline and cortisol rush, if sustained for too long, can deplete your energy, interrupt digestion, affect heart health and stand in the way of your ability to think clearly, to connect with people and to access your higher cognitive functioning. This can fuel a mindset of chronic anxiety and worry, which blocks happiness.

Anxiety can cause different reactions. It can freeze you to the spot like a deer in the headlights, cause you to go mentally blank, lead to indecisiveness and 'analysis paralysis' or leave you feeling chronically exhausted.

Chronic anxiety can turn testosterone's strength into a chronic fight response, with a tendency towards high irritability and blind rage. It can turn dopamine's fluidity and agility into a chronic flight response perhaps from responsibility and commitment or into escapist, addictive behaviours. Chronic anxiety can also turn oxytocin's warmheartedness into feelings like separation anxiety, loneliness and social isolation or push you to overextend yourself in the service of others and end up burnt out. Calming down anxiety is often the key to entering back into your feel-good flow.

Targeting Anxiety

Because chronic anxiety is to blame for so much of our stress, it is worthwhile having a soothing toolkit in mind for calming effect. The techniques offered throughout this book can be of assistance and here are a few examples of on-the-spot tactics working through different bio-chemical qualities:

- ⚙ **Serotonin's grounding quick option:** Centre yourself by standing or sitting evenly over both feet and hips and take a take 5 deep and even breaths.
- ⚙ **Testosterone's strength quick option:** Stand tall and proud, signalling to your brain that you can defeat your anxiety, or be bigger than it, or act despite it.

- ✿ **Oxytocin's warmhearted quick option:** Place a hand on your chest and absorb the warmth from your hand for at least 10 seconds. Add a small smile as you send a heartfelt wish towards yourself, someone else or your circumstance. Or actually reach out for some heartfelt connection or conversation with someone dear.

- ✿ **Dopamine's fluidity or agility quick option:** Shake out your body with the intention of releasing your tensions. You can also consider the positive in your situation and identify even one step forward or one action that you can take that feels helpful and motivating.

Client Story

Shaking Off Anxious Energy to Help With Sleep at Night

Jesse would fall asleep fine, but would wake at 3 a.m. in the clutches of anxiety and not be able to fall back to sleep. Throughout his childhood he was intimidated and bullied, so anxiety was his frequent companion whenever he felt under pressure in his life.

I suggested that the next time Jesse woke at 3 a.m. he should try exploring lying in bed and allowing the energy of his anxiety to shudder through him in the ways that it seemed to 'want' to. He did so and noticed that sometimes it felt as though it was escaping through his head, other times through his arms and often ending with jitters in his legs, which he encouraged to be released through his toes. This shuddering and shaking off of nervous system activation, which is how anxiety can manifest on a physical level, felt satisfying for Jesse. He did wonder initially, however, if all this movement would keep him awake rather than help him fall back to sleep. Yet, without fail, after a few minutes of shuddering and shaking off anxious energy, he felt significantly relieved. I also showed him a series of calming and emotionally containing self-holding techniques. Jesse came to find that he needed these as a final step to help him settle back to sleep. He liked to use the 'over and under' self-hug first, placing right hand under left armpit and left hand on the outside of the right upper arm for a few moments. He followed this with the sleep-support sequence, holding a few different areas from head down to legs for a few moments in turn. Often a big yawn would appear at some stage during the process and he was able to settle into a comfortable position and fall back to sleep.

Jesse also found that upping his regular daily exercise routine to include half an hour to an hour just about every day or three times a week, at least, was also key to keeping his anxiety at bay. He used a mixed exercise practice – running some days, walking other days and some mornings doing some yoga poses in his living room. He still felt anxious at times, but knowing that he could shake off anxiety and soothe himself with self-holding was relieving.

A 3-Step Process for Shaking Off the Energy of Anxiety

This dopamine-stimulating technique of shaking off anxious energy can work well to dissipate anxious energy. You could also use it any time your energy feels worked up, such as when you might feel angry, irritable or restless. Trembling and shaking are natural ways that your nervous system releases energy in order to return to homeostastis. You might have experienced a passing shudder through your body perhaps for no apparent reason or perhaps in response to a passing thought or feeling. You can also tremble with fear or shock and shiver from cold. When you allow or encourage this trembling, shivering and shaking to run its course, which can sometimes take just a minute or two in the case of anxiety, it can allow your nervous system to release energy that might otherwise build up as tension inside you.

- **Step 1: Where do you feel it in your body?** Identify the source area as where your unsettled or agitated feelings seem to originate in your body, for example, in your solar plexus, belly, chest, throat or wherever feels true for you. You might find that taking a few deep breaths can help you to locate this place more easily.
- **Step 2: How does your body want to release?** Feel into which way the energy 'wants' to shudder naturally through and out of your body, such as through the crown of your head, or your hands and fingers, or feet or even your tail bone as endpoints of your body through which energy can release. Invite your body to shake or shudder out the energy through any of these energetic endpoints. Following where the energy feels like it wants to move is key here. When you follow how your body feels like it wants to shudder and shake off energy it can be more effective than deliberately shaking random body parts. Repeat as many times as you need to, feeling the source and then releasing by shuddering or shaking energy out through your endpoints. You can support this if you wish by stretching out arms or legs as you flick or shake off energy.
- **Step 3: Encourage settling.** For this a few deep breaths might do the trick and you can support deeper relaxation with some self-supportive touch, such as a hand to your heart or one hand on your heart, the other cradling your head for a few moments. Or you can use one of the sequences offered, such as the one offered in the chapter on sleep support.

You can use this practice any time of day or night for some welcome nervous system relief. Your stress response also usually ties in with emotional stories about your life. So as you go about this kind of physical release, you may need to acknowledge the triggering event and imagine shaking off the feelings that go along with the event, as you shake off the excess nervous system activation or anxiety.

A Nerve that Plays a Central Role in Both Stress and Happiness

The nervous system offers us one tangible way to measure and track both happiness and stress. It can also give us a physical reference point to help us identify our particular needs for bouncing back from stress. A nerve that is particularly helpful in this regard, as it plays a central and influential role, is the vagus nerve. The vagus nerve is central to your calming, restorative parasympathetic nervous system. It has been referred to as a 'wandering nerve' because of how it snakes through the centre of your body and extends to touch into all of your vital organs from brain to gut. The vagus nerve has two pathways, the ventral and dorsal vagal pathway. Information travels along these pathways in opposite directions to influence our heart, lungs and digestive tract. Happiness is associated with a well-toned ventral vagal pathway.

2 Stress Pathways in the Nervous System

1. **Freeze and collapse:** These stress or survival responses make use of the depressing, downward moving dorsal vagal pathway in response to severe or life-threatening danger. The dorsal vagal pathway is responsible for the sinking feeling that we can get from shock, and initiates an energy conservation mode in our bodies that significantly slows down our heart and breathing rate and our metabolism, causing us to hold really still or collapse. We can also get a shot of endorphins, our natural opiates, to numb pain and help us endure life-threatening situations. When we feel chronically depressed it can be a sign of chronic dorsal vagal dominance, usually representing unresolved trauma. This response is also seen in animals when they feign death in life-threatening situations, which is also a type of collapse response that can be likened to our human impulse to try to make ourselves invisible or hide away without making a sound when we do not feel safe. With this kind of stress response, bouncing back involves a kind of waking up and perhaps finding the energy, courage, motivation or inspiration to live life to the full again.

2. **Fight, flight and anxiety:** These stress or survival responses make use of the activating sympathetic nervous system branch as opposed to your calming parasympathetic branch. When you are in fight or flight mode, the vagus nerve is bypassed in favour of the sympathetic nerve pathways, which speed up your heart rate and increase blood supply to your muscles in preparation for action. Anxiety also activates the sympathetic nervous system with heart and possibly thoughts racing too while at the same time freezing you to the spot so that you might feel stuck, or not know what to do or where to go. When you move into action, which gives an outlet to your nervous system energy, anxiety can naturally dissipate or your body might leap into fight or flight, depending on your circumstance.

Your Nervous System and Happiness

The upward-moving ventral vagal pathway is the pathway that we want to tone and it is linked with health and happiness. It wires our heart and brain together as well as connecting to our lungs and facial muscles. We can feel this as warmth from our hearts, ease in our breathing, animation in our faces, kindness and a twinkle in our eyes, a lilting, relaxed quality to our voices, comfort and openness in our posture and a sense of connection with each other. In this state our brain can function optimally, too, with synchronised access to empathy and compassion and all brain regions. Our digestion and internal organs also work best. It is our parasympathetic nervous system's sweet spot for the functions of 'rest, digest and restoration'. Also, from a nervous system perspective, only when we feel safe can we feel truly happy.

The pioneering research of Dr Stephen Porges and his polyvagal theory adds to our understanding of the ventral vagal nerve pathway in relation to its connection with our hearts. His research shows that when the ventral vagal pathway is active we are more open to being kind, friendly, supportive or loving towards each other. The social engagement aspect is such a strong feature of the ventral pathway that Dr Porges refers to it as a *social nervous system* or *social engagement system* because it allows us to experience co-regulation of our nervous systems, which is our ability to support, comfort and motivate each other. All of us might have experienced this when we share our troubles with someone who cares about us or when we find ways to inspire and motivate another.

Dr Porges refers to the ventral vagal pathway as a natural state of health, growth and restoration. It is this nervous system pathway, associated with feeling safe and secure, that can be toned through the practices in this book, especially those that stimulate serotonin, dopamine and oxytocin. Once toned it then goes on to naturally promote and sustain our happiness in return for our efforts.

Some nicknames given to this ventral vagal pathway are:

- ✸ *'Smart vagus'*, for the way that it promotes optimal and integrated functioning of our brain, making us a more intelligent, open-minded version of ourselves.
- ✸ *'Social vagus'*, for the way it eases our ability to be in happy and satisfying connection with each other.
- ✸ *'Compassion nerve'*, for the way it opens our hearts and creates a direct nervous system connection between heart and mind. This means that our mental intelligence can also be heartfelt.

Toning Your Nervous System for Happiness

In order for stress resilience, and ultimately happiness, to be sustainable, a well-toned vagus nerve is key. The tone of your vagus nerve, alternately referred to as vagal tone, is measured through heart rate variability. This refers to the variability between your heart rate, which is intimately connected with your breathing. On inhalation, heart rate speeds up slightly by the influence of the sympathetic nervous system. On exhalation, heart rate slows down a little by the influence of the parasympathetic nervous system, with its central vagus nerve.

So central is the vagus nerve to your body's relaxation response that there was even a term, 'vagusstoff' (translated from German as 'vagus substance') used for many years to refer to the substance released through the stimulation of the vagus nerve and responsible for the relaxation effect. Later this substance became known as acetylcholine. To feel into the effect of acetylcholine, take a deep breath, or yawn and extend your outbreath for as long as you can. Repeat a few times for on-the-spot calming.

The opposite is noradrenaline, released on inhalation to cause your heart rate to speed up. Noradrenaline is in the adrenaline family, but speeds up your heart rate to a lesser extent than adrenaline. Adrenaline energises us more noticeably than noradrenaline to prepare and propel us into action, such as in high stress or exciting situations. To feel into the effect of noradrenaline, Take a deep breath in and hold it for a count of 3–5, then breathe out. Notice how your head might slightly buzz with energy and how your heart rate can pick up a little. Repeat a few times for a quick energy boost.

Higher heart-rate variability between inhalation and exhalation reflects how quickly your nervous system can settle after activation. In simple terms this points to how skilled you are at calming yourself down and keeping calm as you navigate life's ups and downs. The better you are at it, the healthier your vagal tone. High vagal tone is associated with many positive benefits to health, happiness and even longevity.

The practices of this book work in different ways to support healthy vagal tone. For example:

- ✹ **Serotonin:** Meditation is well researched for its beneficial effect on vagal tone, and the grounding practices offered in this book in general are designed to help you remain calmer, clearer and more stress resilient.
- ✹ **Testosterone and dopamine:** Regular physical exercise to keep your body fit, strong, flexible, fluid and agile has also been well researched in terms of supporting healthy vagal tone, provided that you don't overdo it, in which case your sympathetic nervous system and stress responses can take over.
- ✹ **Dopamine:** Playfulness, adventure, fun and focusing on the positives are also a proven way to support healthy vagal tone.
- ✹ **Oxytocin:** Extending loving-kindness towards yourself and others and investing time and energy in your connections with others are also proven ways to stimulate the ventral vagus nerve pathway and improve vagal tone.

Breathing Basics for Relieving Stress and Promoting Vitality

Bringing awareness to your breathing is yet another effective way to positively influence both vagal tone, shift your state of mind and generally help you to feel more in control. At times you might need to calm down, in which case you would draw on extending your exhalations and breathing more deeply. At times you might need to feel energised, assisted by focusing on speeding up your breathing or breathing more deeply. To follow are a few suggestions for you to explore.

To encourage a noticeable mind-body shift it is recommended that you use any of these breathing techniques for at least 30 seconds or 3–10 minutes for greater impact. If you feel light headed at any point, pause your breathing practice and place a hand on top of your head for some grounding, or rest your head in your hands if you can, perhaps on a desk in front of you or on the ground in a child's pose. Then pick up your breathing practice again if you wish.

Increasing mental clarity through breath
Breathe evenly through your nose to a count of 5 on your inbreath and a count of 5 on your outbreath. Keep this up for 2–10 minutes. Or you could use box breathing (all through your

nose), breathing in for a count of 4, holding for 4, breathing out for 4, holding for 4, etc. Repeat for 6–8 rounds or more if you like.

Calming and relaxing

Lengthen your exhale, such as yawning with a long exhale, sighing a few times or breathing in through your nose for a mental count of 4, then hold for a mental count of 6 or 7 and then breathe out through your mouth for a count of 8. You could also hum or sing your favourite tune. Or you could chant the Om (or Aum) sound, repeating this sound for a few minutes to stimulate the healthy ventral vagus nerve pathway.

Energising, uplifting and warming

Take a long deep inhalation through your nose followed by short bursts of blowing the air out a bit at a time through your mouth until all the air is released. Then start again with your deep breath. Repeat 10 times or as many as you need for an energising pick-me-up.

Centring in yourself and boosting vitality by observing natural breathing

Sit in a comfortable position and observe natural breathing for a few minutes, ideally in and out through your nostrils or, if your nose is blocked, you can of course breathe through your mouth. While observing natural breathing you can make it more interesting by:

- Noticing the temperature of the air that is cooler on inhalation and warmer on exhalation.
- Follow your breath some way into your throat and out into the air in front of you.
- Observe how breathing makes parts of your body expand and contract.
- Notice sensations in your body as you breathe, such as focusing on the skin between nose and mouth and noticing the pulse or tingling sensations of life in this small area where your breath is passing over.
- After this simple practice, as you move through your day, you might also insert moments of briefly noticing your natural breathing as a way to remain connected with yourself in this subtly energising way.

Keeping emotions flowing

When you feel emotional try breathing with your feelings, which could mean simply breathing more deeply as you feel your emotions. Keep this up for a few minutes to help your emotions flow, rather than bottling them up inside you. We often hold our breath instinctively when we feel emotional because breathing amplifies emotions, which can make them feel scary. When we hold our breath our emotions are kept at bay. Allowing ourselves to keep on breathing, even if slowly at first, ensures a good oxygen supply to body and brain to help us respond more mindfully and resourcefully.

Two Studies Promoting Breathing for Stress Relief

1. Breathing for Mental Clarity, Good Decision-making and Emotional Stability

A 2012 study carried out by Dr Justin Kennedy invited 80 banking employees, both male and female, to practise evenly paced breathing (such as breathing in for a count of 5 and out for the same) for 10 minutes a day. Using bio-feedback technology, participants wore sensors attached to a computer to give real-time feedback of their brain function and how it changed with even, deeper breathing. After 21 days of regular practise an average of 62 per cent improvement was seen in the brain's functioning in relation to complex decision-making tasks. Decision-making is a function of the prefrontal cortex, which sits behind the forehead. Activity in this area of the brain increased with the breathing practice, and brain function also became more coherent. Coherence refers to many brain areas active at the same time and has been associated with enhanced mental clarity, focus and insight as well as with positive emotions and the experience of emotional stability.

I have offered this even, deeper breathing practice to a number of clients. I have heard many reports of them feeling more in control, better able to cope with daily ups and downs and to think more clearly under pressure when paying attention to evening out their breathing for short pauses, such as for a minute or two, during the day. Some use the practice for 10 minutes in one go at the start of the day, while others draw on it any time, anywhere. I have also heard from clients that they feel better able to organise and manage their time, be more level headed and more able to enjoy quality time with loved ones. These kinds of feelings contribute to a good foundation for happiness that can carry over to helping us weather life's ups and downs.

Breathing evenly as you might while jogging or walking can offer similar results. Then all you need to do is remind yourself at times during the rest of the day to breathe evenly so as to continue to keep your stress responses at bay.

2. The Effectiveness of the 'Om' Sound in Counteracting Stress

The 'Om' sound combines an extended outbreath with your voice. A 2011 study, carried out by Kalyani and colleagues, found that chanting the 'Om' sound had similar positive effects on the vagus nerve and on deactivating the emotional limbic region of our brains as using electrical vagus nerve stimulation. In this study the 'Om' sound was compared to chanting a 'ssss' sound, with the 'Om' sound yielding better results on the vagus nerve. Another study reported in the *International Journal of Yoga* added that the effect of vibrations on the vagus nerve from chanting the 'Om' sound reduced activity in brain areas involved in the fight, flight and freeze response such as the amygdala and also deactivated areas of the brain associated with depression. The increased oxygenation of the blood from this chanting, which is naturally accompanied by deep breathing, also increased feelings of relaxation in the body as a sign of the calming, healthy parasympathetic nervous system becoming more dominant.

Making a Habit of Recognising What Lights You Up

One final recommendation for this chapter, as a regular way to keep your nervous system toned for happiness, is to pay attention as much as you can to moments that light you up. Deb Dana, author of *The Polyvagal Theory in Therapy*, calls it 'feeding yourself a steady diet of glimmers'. A glimmer, as in a glimmer of hope, is Dana's term for anything that warms your heart, comforts or soothes you, or lights you up. In other words, it is anything that activates your ventral vagus, happy, healthy, compassionate and social nerve pathway.

With practise, recognising glimmers can start to come naturally and you can become more masterful too at looking out for or creating these moments to regularly stoke the hearth of your happiness. It might be from something wonderful that happens, or a simple smile from a stranger, or seeing a beautiful flower or a sunset or hearing wonderful news. You can also amplify the experience to maximise the bio-chemical boost. To do so you can pause to really savour the moment, dwelling on the feelings that it stirs up in you for a few seconds longer than you might normally. This practice of noticing when something lights you up can regularly top up your feel-good bio-chemistry and your happiness reserves to support you through life's ups and downs.

Chapter 13

Happy Posture Practices for Work and Life

'You are as young as your spinal column.'

JOSEPH PILATES

This chapter explores the enlivening combination of serotonin's grounding and dopamine's fluidity as the basis for your posture, with practical guidelines for sitting, standing and releasing tension, which you can apply equally at work and throughout your daily life – from grounding to improved mobility, flexibility, adaptability and stress resilience – all from the awareness and dynamic alignment of your skeleton.

Holding yourself upright with muscular tension creates more wear and tear on your body compared with living in better dynamic and fluid postural alignment. The link between mobility, ageing and quality of life has been extensively studied, with mobility regarded as the most relevant physical ability affecting quality of life. Your natural mobility is highest when you are young, but you can keep up flexibility, fluidity and strength well into your senior years. Becoming more fluid in your posture offers you a pervasive, subtle and very accessible way for promoting lifelong mobility.

Posture

You might think that standing up straight with shoulders pulled back, tummy tucked in and head held high, as if you were a soldier, is a sign of good posture. The truth is that this level of rigidity in our body can negatively affect our breathing and our movement, leading over time to discomfort or pain along our spinal column and interference with the optimal functioning of our internal organs. And if your work involves long hours of sitting at a desk or you spend a lot of time sitting in front of a screen, your body will easily fall into patterns of tension or slouching that also can be detrimental to your wellbeing and happiness.

With dynamic balance, you can learn to stack the bones of our body from the ground up in a way that helps your ease of movement and physical comfort. Each body is unique and differs slightly in its alignment, depending on the natural curvature of the spine. Strength exercises, as in the ones earlier in the book, are good for functional strength. But the main aims with the dynamic approach to posture in this particular chapter are firstly to maintain a solid, stabilising relationship with gravity and grounding and then to allow energy to flow freely through your body as you breathe and move through life. This is achieved by aligning your skeleton via a dynamic sense balance. Balance needs to be dynamic because we are never truly still. Even when we are doing nothing, there is movement going on inside of us, such as breathing, heart beating and digestion churning. Life is movement and movement is life.

Accepting this constant movement and working with it can open your mind to think more clearly, optimise the brain functioning and lighten your experience of life. On a physiological level, tuning into dynamic balance can free up the pathways through your body for improved nervous system communication and blood circulation. On a physical level it can facilitate movement through life with minimal wear and tear on bones and soft tissues.

In all, with this more fluid, dynamic approach to uprightness, your muscles will take on a more natural and almost effortless supportive role, which can be enlivening and promote a sense of youthfulness no matter your age.

Sitting Posture: 3-Point Check

1. **Sit with both feet flat on the ground, parallel and with knees hip distance apart:** The ideal is to place both feet flat on the ground, although if you wear heels you can still follow the instructions and work with your heels. Shift forwards a bit on your

seat if you need to so that your knees are slightly lower than hip level. This position allows you to hold your spine upright, which also gently engages your core muscles as opposed to leaning back into your backrest.

2. **Adjust hips to sit centre:** Roll your hips backwards and forwards a few times, rounding and arching into your lower back as you do so, and then find centre so your sitting bones point downwards towards the ground. Your spine through to the crown of your head can naturally seem to float upwards as opposed to having to exert any strain to maintain uprightness.

3. **Press down into your feet:** This engages your thigh muscles and can cause a little lift in your chest area as it also gives a boost to your sense of strength and focus. It is an action that you can repeat any time you wish to achieve this effect.

A Few Notes About Posture

It's not possible to maintain perfect posture all day, but even if you just remind yourself of your happy posture for 2 minutes a few times a day you can train your muscle memory to keep coming back for more of the benefits that this can bring.

If you work at a desk, it can be a good idea to run your quick posture checks before you sit down to work, and each time you return to your desk after breaks. If you do this regularly enough, your body will remind you rather than the other way around. Then you can go on to focus on the work you need to do. Remember there is no need to stress about keeping this exact posture as you move on to work. The whole point is stress relief as well as improved physical comfort and mobility.

Also if you get tired or need back support, use a seat with a comfortable, upright backrest and push your seat in close to your desk so that your spine is upright in the position against your backrest as you sit at your desk.

Stress-relief Options Sitting at Your Desk

Estimated time: minimum of 2 minutes

The following exercises target common areas of tension including your neck, shoulders, arms, hands and back. Choose the exercises that target your areas of tension and you can experiment with each motion, perhaps discovering benefits in many of the exercises and devising your own routine for a 2 minute stress relief break.

Nose Circles to Alleviate Upper Neck Tension

When you feel stressed, it is likely that there is tension in the sub-occipital muscles that attach the skull to the neck, leading to neck tension or pain over time. These muscles work really hard when your neck is held forward or when you're looking down for a period of time, such as when you lock your focus on a computer screen or focus down on your phone or even read a book. This simple exercise can help to ease tension and lubricate your sub-occipital area. You can carry it out with eyes open; for a more mindful experience, close your eyes.

The exercise involves 'drawing' circles in the air with your nose as if your nose has a paint brush extending out from its tip. Move 3 times in one direction and then the other and repeat a few times until your neck feels looser. You can also play with the motion, such as making circles bigger and smaller, spiraling circles inwards and outwards, drawing a figure of 8 with your nose, or exploring free movement of your head and neck joints to loosen up any kinks that you might come across. As you explore freely in this way you might also like to imagine a paintbrush extending upwards from the crown of your head so that your smooth motions can also 'paint on the ceiling'. Keep your shoulders relaxed throughout to avoid building up strain in your neck.

Shoulder Circles

Circle both your shoulders forwards and then backwards a few times and then one at a time in a cycling-like motion. To increase the movement while raising one shoulder at a time, you could play with raising the elbow on the same side as your raised shoulder as if spreading your imaginary wings one at a time. You can also play with other shoulder movements, such as shaking out your shoulders or allowing the rest of your body to follow naturally along with your movements to increase the loosening up effect, or you could explore making your shoulder movements smaller and more focused as you try to isolate your shoulder movements from your spine to unlock tension that can bind your shoulders to your neck and spine.

Side-to-side Swaying

In your sitting position, bring your arms to your sides; if this is difficult in your chair, you can place your hands on your thighs with arms relaxed. Sway your spine from side to side like a reed while remaining evenly seated over both hips. Continue for a minute or two. This subtle swaying movement can focus your awareness on releasing tension and increasing mobility and fluidity in the side-to-side motion of your spinal column. This can go on to support being more centred when upright. You might even notice your spine clicking into better alignment as you do so although you would never force this, only swaying mindfully while inviting your movement to gradually become more fluid, especially through tight areas. To help with this, you can explore initiating the movement from different parts of your torso – waist, lower back, upper back – noticing how some areas of your back are more mobile than others. Allow your neck to follow along with the movement rather than overstretching sideways. When you return to upright on completion of your minute or so of swaying, take a moment to notice how your back feels.

Arm Reaches

Reach both arms upwards and take a deep breath. Then alternate reaching up as high as you can with one arm at a time, repeating a few times. If you wish, move on to playing with free movement of your arms and hands, perhaps snaking them and twisting and turning them to increase your sense of flow and vitality in your arms and upper body.

Hand and finger movements: Your hands also build up tension. Take a few moments to move your fingers as if they were sea anemones with tentacles moving about in water. Include all fingers or move one finger at a time. It can feel good to end by shaking out your hands and arms a little before resuming your work.

Lower Back Support with Hip Walking Side to Side

Focusing on your hip bones, raise one hip slightly off your seat a few times, then the other. If you wish, move into free movement into your lower back area or some gentle shaking out of your hips from side to side before resuming your normal sitting position. For a more subtle option that can also release tension in the lower spine, you can press both feet into the ground a few times and then alternate pressing one foot and then the other down into the ground a few times. As you do so, allow your upper body to relax and be swayed ever so slightly by the motion initiated by pressing into your feet.

Unravel Your Slouch and Energise Your Whole Spine

Whether you slouch or not, this exercise can help to loosen up and energise your fluid uprightness. It works well coordinated with breathing.

- Breathe out as you slouch your body, rounding your spine into a c-curve and allowing your head to follow the movement.
- Breathe in as you unfold your body to upright and into a backward arch, with chin raised slightly upwards.

✺ Repeat a few times, encouraging all vertebrae to participate in this fluid undulation. Notice how some parts of your spine might slouch and arch easily and others might feel more stuck or less bending. As you play with these movements, you can experience your spine freeing up – something that also improves with time and practise. The flow of this motion can leave you feeling quite energised in your whole spine.

✺ Find centre again, with your sitting bones pointing downwards. Then return to your work with no more slouching!

Note About Ergonomics

Ergonomics is the study of our efficiency in our work environment that includes, for example, desk height, chair features, computer screen and keypad distance as well as the orientation of our computation to us. These can all make a difference to our comfort, energy levels and productivity at work. For example, if your seat is too high so that your feet cannot reach the floor, it is a good idea to invest in a lower one with greater ergonomic utility. Or if you notice a lot of shoulder, neck or arm tension, you might consider the height of your desk and the ease of your reach to a computer keyboard that could improve your comfort, energy efficiency and productivity.

Standing Posture 4-Point Check

1. **Place both feet flat on the ground, legs parallel and hip distance apart:** Work around whatever shoes you have on.

2. **Shift your weight slightly back over your heels:** This helps with spinal alignment and stability. If you like you can imagine a long dinosaur-like tail extending down to balance from your tail bone down to the ground.

3. **Unlock your knees:** This is an important step because tension in your knees limits freedom of movement. Loosen your knee joint just enough to be able to feel the ground through your feet and walk easily. To maintain optimal mobility, avoid locking your knees as you go on to the next step of stacking your spine.

4. **Stack your spine from the ground up:** Drop your weight down into the ground through your feet and allow the bones of your spine to naturally stack from the ground up until your spine balances lightly in uprightness from feet up to head. In this position you are in touch with gravity through your feet, particularly your heels, which root down into the ground and you are in touch with levity as your head might seem to float upwards on top of your spine.

Exercises for Happy Posture While Standing

The following exercises can be practised any time and anywhere, discreetly while waiting in the shopping line or you can make bigger movements when in private.

Stand Into One Foot at a Time

This can create a small sway from side to side as you shift your weight over one foot and then the other. To assist with this sway, press down into the foot you are standing into to assist your shifting over to the other foot. Keep your weight slightly back over your heels as you do so. Allow the rest of your body to relax and follow along with the subtle side-to-side sway. To end, centre over both your feet.

Play With a Stepping Motion to Bring Greater Ease of Movement

You might raise your knees one at a time as if slowly walking or marching on the spot (or actually move around if you like or play with your freedom of motion while out and about too). You can also add a few extras like arm motions that cycle naturally with each step, opposite arm and leg moving together and inviting your shoulders and arms to move freely and loosely. If you are able to, you might play some music if it feels helpful. Ground well through your feet and stack your posture from the ground up continuously as you play freely with the fluidity of your movement too.

Unravel Your Slouch While Standing

- ✺ Breathe out and allow your body to fold forwards as much as you like over bent legs.
- ✺ Breathe in and unfold your body from the ground up (pressing down into your feet, heels in particular, and then unfolding and stacking your spine) to return to upright. Invite your muscles to remain relaxed throughout as they learn to support rather than control your uprightness. Repeat 5–10 times.
- ✺ Finally, move freely any way you like.

Make Time to be Fluid and Grounded in Your Posture Each Day

Using whichever of this chapter's practices that you feel drawn to at the time, pause now and again each day, even if just for 30 seconds or a couple of minutes when you can, to plug into your grounded fluidity through posture. This can prevent tension from building up in your body, build up your stress resilience and wake up the energy of positivity. With time you will also become more skilled at catching moments of postural tension and intervening with some grounding and fluid movement to restore the optimal, dynamic posture that promotes your happiness.

*Helpful Workout Recommendation
GROUNDED AND FLUID POSTURE WORKOUT

To turn the exercises of this chapter into a full workout, go through them in sequence, starting with the sitting or standing practices, as you prefer, and the posture checks, then moving on to the fluid movements of various kinds and ending by returning to a few moments of centring and settling in dynamic postural alignmentP

Grounded and Fluid Posture

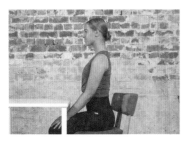

Sitting posture.

Nose circles.

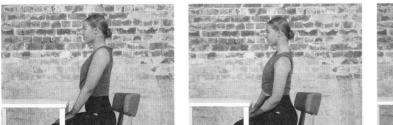 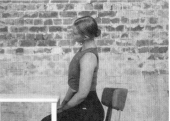

SHOULDER CIRCLES: Both shoulders together forwards and backwards and cycling shoulders.

Side-to-side swaying.

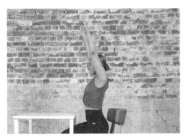 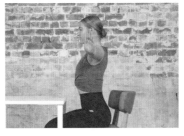 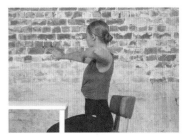

Arm reaches and free arm movement.

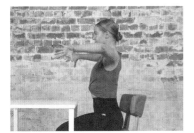 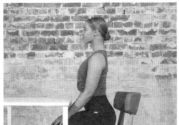 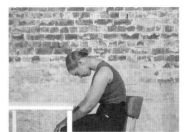

Hand and finger movements.

Arch and round spine to unravel slouching.

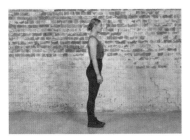 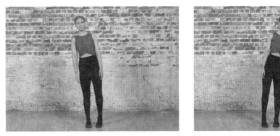

Standing posture

Weight from foot to foot, then centre and ground through both feet.

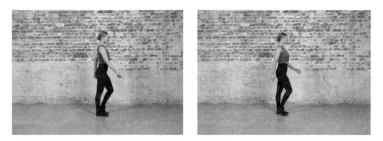

Play with stepping motion to encourage freedom of movement.

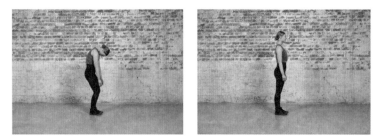

UNRAVEL SLOUCH WHILE STANDING: Round and lengthen spine, stacking posture from ground up.

Happiness Boosting Menu and Quick Reference Guide

This appendix contains all the practices in this book with page numbers as a quick reference guide. This helps you to see all the practices, choose what you are drawn to at the time, flag new practices to try out at different times and follow the recommendations or challenges to boost and sustain your happiness. To start with there is also a list of the three brief self-assessments offered in the book that can help orient you to most relevant practices.

Quick Tips for a Sense of the Bio-chemistry of Happiness

- Page 10: Quick tips to get the serotonin feeling
- Page 11: Quick tips to get the oxytocin feeling
- Page 12: Quick tips to get the dopamine feeling
- Page 14: Quick tips to get the testosterone feeling
- Page 15: Quick tips to get the endorphin feeling
- Page 17: Quick tip to get the cortisol, stress-hormone feeling

Three Self-Assessment Opportunities to Identify Which Happy Chemicals to Boost at This Time

The Physical Skills of Happiness

Grounding to Boost the Serotonin Experience of Happiness

Strength to Boost the Testosterone Experience of Happiness

Fluidity, Agility and Flexibility to Boost the Dopamine Experience of Happiness

Warmheartedness to Boost the Oxytocin Experience of Happiness

Bouncing Back From Stress and Toning Your Nervous System for Happiness

Happy Posture Practices for Work and Life

Workout Menu

All workout guides, except for the 'Grounded and Fluid Posture Workout', which is in the 'Happy Posture' chapter, are contained in Appendix 2 at the end of the book.

Support Following Workouts

(ALSO IN APPENDIX 2)

Page 213: A few stretches and muscle-recovery suggestions.

Bouncing Back From Stress - a Reference Chart

PHYSICAL STRESS RESPONSE	SOME POSSIBLE CORRESPONDING EMOTIONS OR FEELINGS	RECOMMENDED FOCUS
Fight Response (Sympathetic nervous system activation)	• Anger • Rage • Annoyance or frustration • Irritability • Agitation • Burnout • Grandiosity • Wanting to hurt yourself or others	Calm your nervous system with serotonin's grounding and oxytocin's warmheartedness practices. Then find healthy ways to channel strength, such as physical exercise and being ambitious.

Flight Response (Sympathetic nervous system activation)	• Restlessness • Fear • Panic • Feeling jittery • Boredom • Non-commitment • Thinking or speaking a mile a minute • Wanting to escape or run away such as with escapist or addictive behaviour	Calm your nervous system with serotonin's grounding and oxytocin's warmheartedness practices. Then find healthy ways to channel restlessness, such as physical exercise and keeping up exciting goals.
Anxious freeze response (Sympathetic nervous system activation)	• Anxiety • Relentless worry • Shame with anxiety • Over-thinking • Low self-esteem • Rumination • Analysis paralysis • Stage fright with high anxiety • Social anxiety • Performance anxiety	Calm your nervous system with serotonin's grounding and oxytocin's warmheartedness practices. Then, in baby steps, step into testosterone's courage and dopamine's risk-taking to help you achieve all you want to in life.
Out of balance 'tend and befriend' response (Sympathetic nervous system activation as compared to healthy 'tend and befriend' response, which uses the healthy ventral vagal, social engagement nervous system when we actively give our support to others)	• Martyrdom • Burnout or compassion fatigue	Calm your nervous system with serotonin's grounding and oxytocin's warmheartedness practices. Then keep up with self-care as you extend out to others.

Out of balance 'cry or call for help' response (Sympathetic nervous system activation. The 'cry for help' response is a natural, healthy way to draw on our social support networks when we need to. Babies literally cry for attention or help. As we grow older this can turn into calling for or seeking out help in other ways than crying. Calling or asking for help can express healthy access to our ventral vagal, social engagement nervous system unless our reliance on others is anxiety ridden, in which case it can switch into sympathetic activation)	• Desperation • Separation anxiety • Crying easily • Acting out for attention • Fear of being alone • Anxious sense of abandonment • Anxious reliance on others to the detriment of self-sufficiency • Fear of asking for help • Yearning or pining for a special person • Spiritual yearning perhaps for guidance, direction or to know our true purpose	Soothe your nervous system with serotonin's grounding and oxytocin's warmheartedness practices. In the longer term, build up your testosterone-related inner strength and stay connected with what inspires and excites you for dopamine-related energy and personal motivation.
Numb, dissociated or blank freeze response (Parasympathetic dorsal vagal branch)	• Empty • Lost • Confused • Stuck • Withdrawn • Emotionally numb • Mentally blank or foggy • Disorientated • Feeling like you can't find your voice or words • Dreamy • Stage fright with blankness • Over-intellectualising	Energise your nervous system with dopamine's fluidity, agility and flexibility and testosterone's strength practices, starting with whichever you are drawn to first. Then in the longer term develop a healthy relationship with serotonin's grounding for stress resilience and invest in warmheartedness too to perhaps assist with emotional healing.

Collapse response (Parasympathetic dorsal vagal branch. Of course, if we actually collapse or faint from stress we do not feel anything. The possible corresponding emotions refer to a more subtle, chronic expression of collapse response when a part of us feels collapsed or locked away inside while we might go on with daily living)	• Depression • Shame with melancholy • Melancholy • Helplessness • Hopelessness • Giving up • Loneliness • Isolation • Feeling all alone in the world • Not wanting to be here	Gently encourage your nervous system to wake up and be in connection with others and the world through serotonin-related grounding practices and oxytocin-related warmheartedness. Then when you feel ready, move on to connecting with the higher energy of dopamine's fluidity, agility and flexibility and the courage of testosterone-related strength practices.

Notes About Using This Reference Chart

The list of emotions that match physical stress responses is not a comprehensive list; rather, it is a list of common complaints that I have come across. Also, you do not need to identify with all of the feelings on the list. Even if you just identify with one way of feeling or emotion, you can apply the relevant stress-relief technique (either calming or energising). You might also recognise a combination of emotions or feelings that cross over between the need for calming and energising. Use the one that feels most helpful in the moment. There are also complex and potentially extremely challenging emotional experiences such as grief, trauma and psychiatric disorders. In these cases use the techniques that work best for you and that best match how you feel in the moment, for some relief. This can be empowering to some extent, but it will be necessary for you to seek appropriate professional support for a comprehensive treatment plan.

Challenges

Regular Daily Challenge Options

- ✷ Use your favourite short practice or quick tip now and again daily.
- ✷ Use a short practice or quick tip that you know you need to develop even if you don't particularly like it.

3-Day Challenge

Use your favourite short practice or quick tip from this book, and repeat once or twice a day for 3 days. This can be long enough to log the technique in your mind, making you more likely to think of applying it in future at a time when it might be helpful. Repeat the 3-day challenge as many times as you like with any other techniques that you are curious to become familiar with.

7-Day Challenges

- **Bouncing back from stress:** Refer to the chapter on bouncing back from stress and toning your nervous system for happiness and apply appropriate stress-management techniques daily, maybe once or twice a day, to hone your stress-management skills.
- **Focus on breathing:** Dedicate a week to growing your awareness of your breathing to explore what value this might bring. Find regular opportunities to apply practices from 'Breathing basics for relieving stress and promoting vitality' offered in the stress chapter.
- **Build happy posture familiarity:** Find a couple of opportunities daily for a week to apply some of the practices from the Happy Posture chapter, spending a few minutes at a time growing your familiarity with their value.

21-Day Challenge

- Invest in building one of the physical skills of happiness for 21 days. Choose the one that you feel you could benefit from most at the time. It is recommended that you make daily use of your choices from the short practice and quick tip options pertaining to the skill that you are developing, perhaps inserting them in gaps in your day. It is also recommended that you make use of the relevant workout/s, if you are physically able to, carrying out one workout per day for at least 3 days per week over the 3-week period. All of this ensures that you stimulate and reinforce the skill on a daily basis for the 21 days.
- Journalling your progress can be interesting if you are open to doing so, or you are welcome to represent how you feel in any artistic method of your preference. It can be interesting to pay attention to what might open up in your life during this time of developing the particular skill.

Create Your Own Challenge!

You are most welcome to design your own challenge or share a challenge with a friend or group, then you could discuss your progress, support each other and also hold each other accountable to the challenge.

7 ILLUSTRATED WORKOUT GUIDES AND SUPPORT FOR MUSCLE RECOVERY

These easy-to-follow exercise routines range from 10–30 minutes and are adaptable to different levels of fitness and flexibility.

Workouts

1. Grounding workout with short meditation
2. Bedtime workout for unwinding towards peaceful sleep
3. Self-holding sequence to relax for sleep
4. Strength workout
5. Workout for boosting creativity and zest for life
6. Workout for strengthening your reach and perseverance
7. Heart-opening workout

Support following workouts

A few stretches and muscle-recovery suggestions.

Preparing For a Workout

- Allow up to half an hour of uninterrupted time to carry out your chosen workout. Any time of day will do, except for the workout at bedtime.
- Wear comfortable, loose-fitting clothing or stretchy exercise gear.
- The workouts can be carried out inside in a carpeted area, or on a yoga mat or outside if you prefer and are able. So long as you can extend your arms and legs out in each direction, that should be enough space.
- Have a cushion available for sitting positions and occasionally for lying down too for added support.
- The strength Workout has the option to include dumbbells (not essential). If you wish to raise something weighty, you could even use full, 2-litre milk bottles or a bag full of groceries! Be creative.
- There is also the option in the strength workout of holding a piece of string or skipping rope long enough to be held and stretched between your hands when your arms are raised above your head.

Important Notes About Using the Workouts

- With all exercises, never work into pain. If you feel pain during a workout, back off and perhaps explore slowing your movement down or finding an alternate pathway for your movement that is comfortable.
- If you feel pain, it is important to consult with a medical professional or physiotherapist before proceeding with any self-treatment or exercise at home.
- Especially if you have an existing physical injury or medical condition, it is important to consult with your health-care provider or specialist before trying out new exercises.
- Always listen to your body and work within your range of capability while carrying out the exercises to take best care of yourself.

Exercises to Promote Grounding and Serotonin's Serene, Stable and Expansive Happiness

'Get yourself grounded and you can navigate even the stormiest roads in peace.'

STEVEN GOODIER

There are two workouts offered here to promote grounding. One is a grounding workout Mnviting you to strengthen your legs, your stability and balance over your legs and your ability to surrender your weight into gravity, also supported at the end by the inclusion of a short meditation practice. You are invited to use each exercise as an opportunity to feel grounded through your hips, legs and feet while exploring how your upper body and your uprightness engage to support your physcial stability.

The other is a bedtime workout to support a good sleep at night – fundamental to our ability to feel grounded. This includes a series of relaxing exercises designed for letting go of tension in key areas of your body so that you can more easily relax into peaceful sleep.

Grounding Workout With Short Meditation

Time estimate: 15-20 minutes

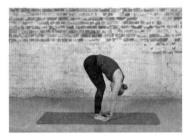

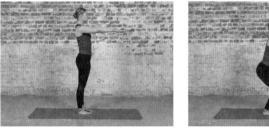

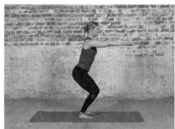

1. Hang forwards over slightly bent legs, feet hip distance apart and parallel. Hold for 5 breaths.

2. SQUATS: Arms parallel to ground. Feet hip distance apart and parallel. Inhale standing, exhale squatting. Repeat 8 times. Increase intensity by moving slower, to a count of 3, into and out of squat.

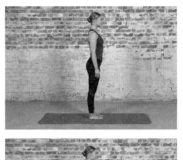
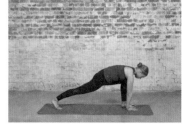
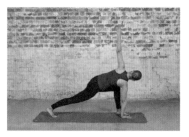

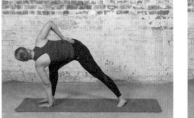

3. LUNGE WITH TWIST SEQUENCE:

Start standing. Exhaling step right foot forwards, bending knee and placing hands alongside foot.

Inhaling twist, raising right arm up and looking up. Exhaling return hand alongside foot. Then inhale stepping right foot back alongside left in standing position.

Repeat sequence to the left. Repeat 3 times each side.

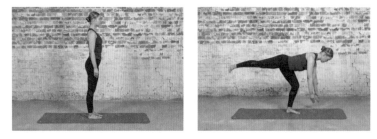

4. SIDEWAYS LUNGE WITH REACH: Start with legs fairly wide apart, feet flat on the ground. Bend right knee and reach right hand to ground in front of left foot. Switch sides so left hand touches ground in front of right foot. Repeat from side to side 4-6 times.

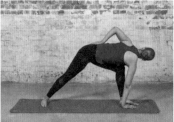

5. FORWARD LUNGE WITH BALANCE: Start standing. Step forward onto slightly bent right leg. Find balance as raise left leg behind you with foot flexed. Arms reach downwards. Hold for 3 slow breaths then step back to standing. Repeat to left. Repeat 3 times each side.

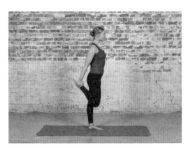

6. THIGH STRETCH WHILE STANDING:
Hold for 3 breaths each side.

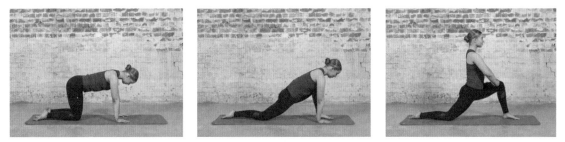

7. LUNGE STRETCH; Start on all fours; step right foot forward between hands, knee bent at a right angle as ease into lunge. Feel stretch across front of left hip. If you can, bring hands onto knees. Hold for 3-5 breaths. Then repeat on the other side.

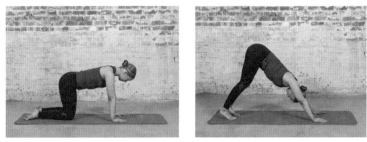

8. DOWNWARD-FACING DOG STRETCH: Start on all fours. Curl toes under and raise hips high, easing chest down between arms and extending legs as much as you can with heels pressing down towards the ground. Hold for 5 breaths. Then walk hands towards feet.

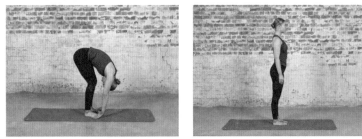

9. HANG FORWARDS: Hang forwards over slightly bent legs before unfolding to standing.

**For a more intensive workout:
Repeat entire grounding workout 2 or 3 more times before moving on to meditation.**

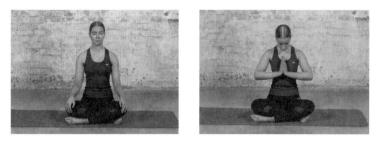

10. 5-10 MINUTE MEDITATION: Sit in upright, comfortable position on a cushion. Hands over knees or on thighs, palms down. Eyes closed preferably or focus down on the ground.

- Observe 10 natural breaths focusing on breath entering and leaving nose or filling and emptying body.
- Scan body from head to toe, pausing briefly to feel sensations in each area. End by holding awareness for a few moments in body as a whole.
- On a long exhalation make a foghorn-like 'vuuuuu' sound. Repeat 3 times.
- Bow to close your meditation, hands in prayer pose.

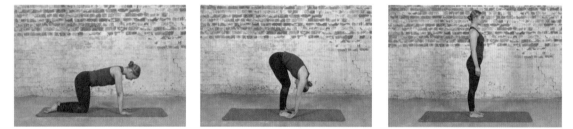

11. To return to standing move through all fours to hang forwards over legs for a few breaths and then unfold your spine smoothly up to standing.

Bedtime workout for unwinding towards peaceful sleep

Time estimate: 15 minutes

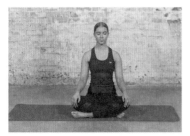

1. 3 SLOWING-DOWN BREATHS: Sit comfortably and make each in and out breath even and longer than the one before.

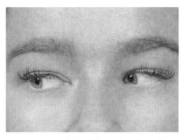

2. EYE ROLLS: End focusing for a few breaths on a point on the ground with soft eyes.

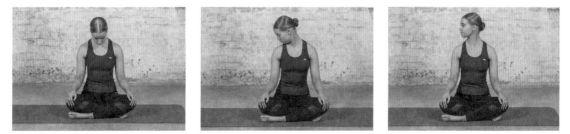

3. HEAD ROLLING FROM SIDE TO SIDE: Exhaling lower chin to chest then inhaling move and raise chin to the right so you are looking over your right shoulder. Exhaling lower chin down to chest again and inhale raising head to the left. Repeat 3 times each side.

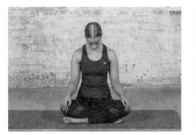

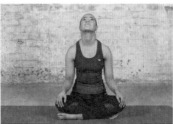

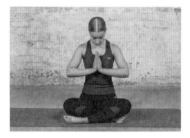

4. Exhaling, lower your head, inhaling raise your head. Repeat 3 times.

5. Bow head towards hands in prayer pose. Hold for 3 breaths feeling stretch to back of neck.

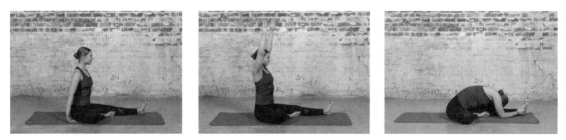

6. FORWARD BEND OVER ONE LEG: Sitting, extend right leg and bend left leg bringing left foot in to touch side of right leg. Inhaling raise arms sideways and up. Exhaling reach into forward bend over right leg, head towards knee, taking hold where you can (ankle or foot). Hold for 3-5 breaths. Then reverse motion to return to upright sitting position. Repeat to left.

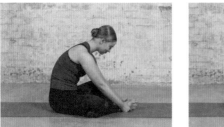
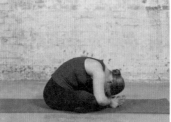
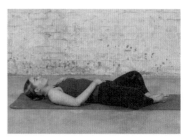

7. Butterfly legs with feet together a comfortable distance away from you. Briefly massage legs from hips to toes. Then relax forwards elbows over knees, head relaxing towards feet. Hold for 3-5 breaths. Then unfold spine to upright.

8. Legs in butterfly, lie down on back. Place one hand over chest, the other over lower belly. Hold for 5 easy breaths.

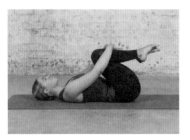
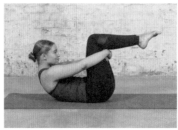

9. Hug knees in over belly. Hold for 3 breaths.

10. ROLLING BALL: Tuck chin in to chest, hook hands under knees and roll backwards and forwards a few times for a massage to your spine.

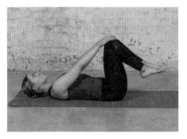
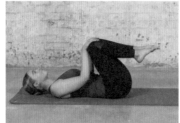
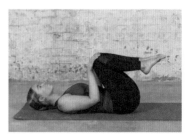

11. Lie flat on your back, hands to knees. Inhaling, move knees away as far as arms allow. Exhaling hug knees in over belly. Repeat 3 times slowly

12. Holding knees, draw 3 circles in the air in each direction with knees for massage to lower back. End hugging knees over belly.

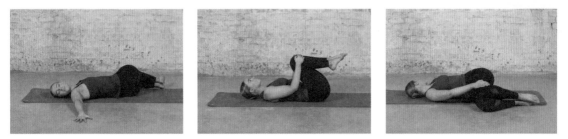

13. SPINAL TWIST: With knees hugged in over belly, hold right hand over left knee and ease legs over to right towards the ground. Extend left arm out to left side, palm flat, and look to left. Hold for 3 breaths. Return to hug knees and repeat to left. End hugging knees for 2 deep breaths.

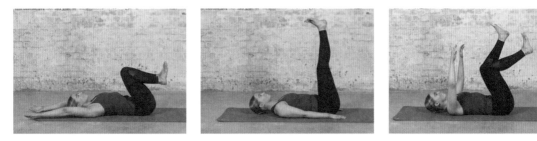

14. LEG RAISES: Inhaling, bend knees, flex feet and raise arms alongside head. Exhaling extend legs upwards, raising flexed feet and lowering arms to sides. Repeat 3 times slowly.

15. Shake out arms and legs while lying on your back.

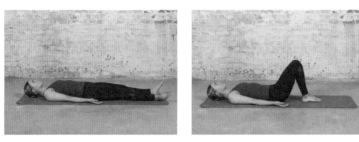

16. Lie flat on your back for a few minutes of complete rest. If you wish to support lower back, bend knees with feet flat on ground.

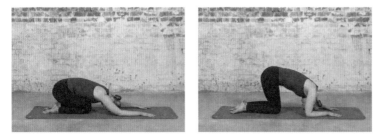

17. HEAD MASSAGE: From lying on back, curl onto side and move into child's pose with forehead on ground and arms alongside head. Then roll forwards and backwards a few times over your head for a gentle head massage. End in child's pose for a deep breath.

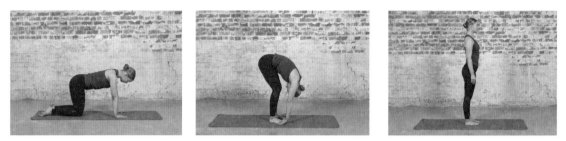

18. Transition to standing by moving through all fours then hanging forwards over bent legs for a few moments and then unfolding spine to upright.

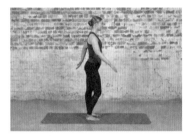

19. Shake out your body from head to toe for final tension release then make your way to bed.

Self-holding sequence to relax for sleep (while lying down)

Hold each position for at least 30 seconds breathing naturally

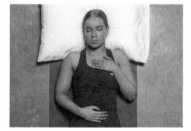

1. Both hands hold on top of head.

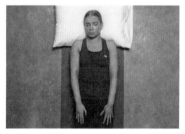

2. One hand forehead, other hand behind neck.

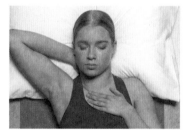

3. One hand forehead, other hand chest.

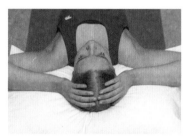

4. One hand chest, other hand lower belly.

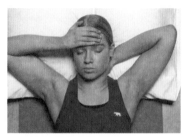

5. Both hands on thighs.

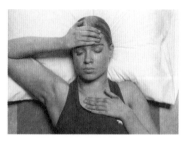

6. One hand behind neck, other hand on chest.

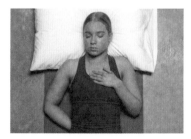

7. OPTIONAL EXTRA: One hand under tail bone, other hand on chest.

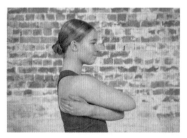

FOR USE ANY TIME: Over-under self-hug (right hand under left arm holding side of chest, left hand over right) for emotional containment and self-soothing.

Exercises to Promote Strength and Testosterone's Confident, Determined and Ambitious Kind of Happiness

'Strength does not come from winning. Your struggles develop your strength. When you go through hardships and decide not to surrender, that is strength.'

ARNOLD SCHWARZENEGGER

This workout is designed to build your physical and functional strength. Functional strength is the kind of strength that supports the actions of your daily lives, such as walking, lifting shopping bags, carrying children, bending and stretching to pick up and reach for objects, sitting down, standing up and the like. The intention is to make your daily activities easier to perform and help to prevent injury while developing your inner strength and confidence to achieve your goals and stand up for yourself in life.

Functional exercises involve many muscle groups at once, as opposed to isolating muscles. This is because our daily movements require the coordination of many muscle groups working together. Daily movements also require a coordinated working relationship between the brain and nervous system, which gives the commands. Exercises that isolate muscles – such as sit ups, bicep curls or leg extensions – are helpful at times but can be less effective than training our body in a coordinated, holistic way, especially in the long run. One example is the difference between squats that work many muscle groups at once and knee extensions that isolate leg muscles. Squats are usually more effective in supporting our ability to stand up from a seated position or bend to pick up something heavy, compared to isolated knee extensions. Squats, therefore, have a greater 'transfer effect'. Good functional strength is what we want to maintain throughout our lives to feel stronger, more secure and more in control of our bodies.

Core strength is really important for our sense of strength and stability. From a functional strength perspective, the core is naturally strengthened in an integrated way when we target many different muscle groups at once during exercise. For a sense of engaging just the right amount of core strength, try finding your balance on one leg. Or you could align your posture well and notice how core muscles are naturally activated to support you in a way that you can feel your feet on the ground while standing tall. This type of core exercise is not the same as holding your belly in more tightly, which you might do due to social pressure; this type of stance, however, simply limits your ability to breathe fully and feel grounded.

To feel strong, you do want to power up your upper body. With the functional exercises included in the following workout, you can grow upper-body strength in an integrated way using the rest of your body. This can help you to stand tall and feel good about yourself as well as helping you with daily chores like carrying shopping bags.

Strength Workout

Time estimate: 20 minutes

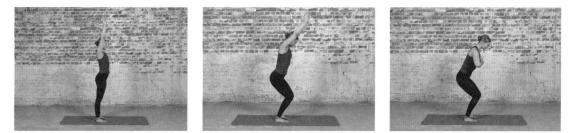

1. Squat with arms raised, palms facing in or holding string or stick between hands for support. Inhaling upright, exhaling into squat. Move slowly, to mental count of 3 in and out of squat. Carry out 6-8 squats. Increase intensity by holding dumbbells together at chest level for squats.

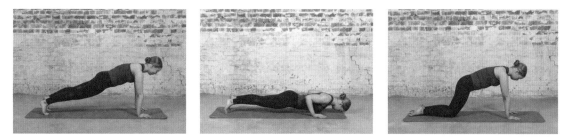

2. 8-16 push ups, inhaling as push up, exhaling as lower down. If needed, place knees on ground.

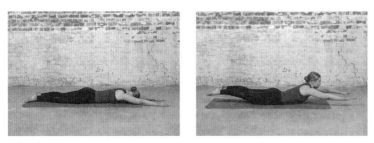

3 SUPERMAN FLYING POSE: Start lying face down on ground with arms extended alongside head on ground. Inhale raising upper body and legs off ground and looking forwards (like Superman flying). Exhale lowering to ground. Repeat 6-8 times.

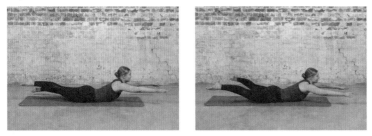

4. Holding Superman flying position, kick legs for a count of 8 (like swimming freestyle) while looking forwards. Alternate with opening and closing arms and legs 4 times. Repeat 3 times.

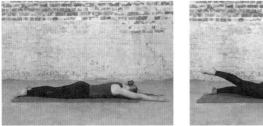
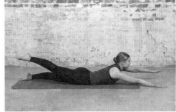

5. OPPOSITE ARM AND LEG RAISES: Lie face down. Inhaling raise right arm and left leg while looking down to ground. Exhaling lower. Repeat raising left arm and right leg. Repeat 6-8 times.

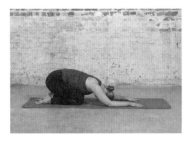
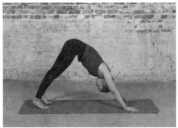

6. Rest in child's pose for 8 relaxing breaths with arms resting alongside head.

7. DOWNWARD-FACING DOG STRETCH: Move through all fours into a downward-facing dog position, raising hips high and pressing down through hands and heels. Hold for 5 breaths.

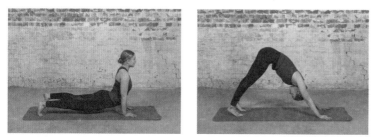

8. UPWARD- AND DOWNWARD-FACING DOG STRETCH: Inhaling lower hips to just above ground, raising head to look up in upward-facing dog stretch. Exhaling raise hips and press down through hands and heels into downward-facing dog stretch. Repeat 6-8 times.

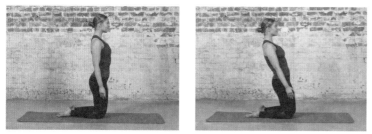

9. KNEELING BACK ON KNEES: Start kneeling with legs slightly apart and parallel. Inhaling sit upright, exhaling lean back aiming for straight line from knees to head. Repeat 8 times.

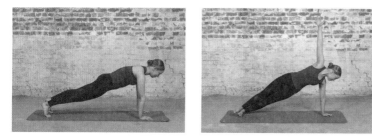
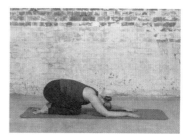

10. PLANK WITH TWIST: Start in plank position. Inhale raising right arm upward as body twists to right. Look down to bottom hand. Right foot naturally moves on top of left. Exhale returning to plank pose. Repeat to left then repeat 4-6 times alternating sides

11. Rest in child's pose for 8 relaxing breaths with arms resting alongside head.

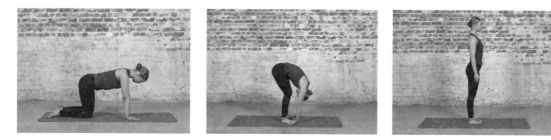

12. Transition to standing by moving through all fours then hanging forwards over bent legs for a few moments and then unfolding spine to upright with head coming up last.

The following 3 exercises are optional if you have dumbbells, otherwise move on to Warrior 1.

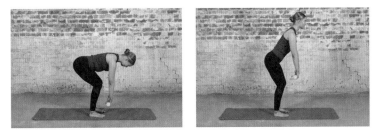

13. OPTIONAL DEADLIFTS WITH DUMBBELLS: Standing, hold dumbbell in each hand and lean forwards so dumbbells at ankle level. Keep spine extended, tail bone reaching backwards and weight back on heels. Inhaling raise upper body so dumbbells rise to thigh level with knees bent, exhaling lower back down. Repeat 8 times.

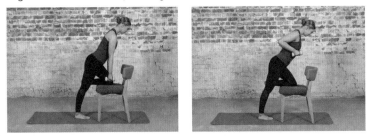

14. STANDING PULL-UPS WITH DUMBBELL: Lean your knee on a seat, holding dumbbell in right hand hanging down at your side. Raise and lower 8 times. Switch sides and repeat.

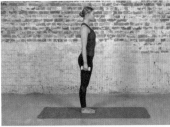
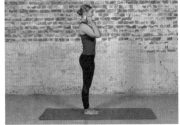
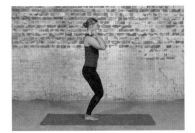

15. STANDING DUMBBELL PRESS-UP: Hold a dumbbell in each hand at your sides. Raise dumbbells to top of shoulders then bend knees, and as extending legs raise dumbbells up high. Repeat 8 times.

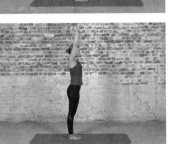

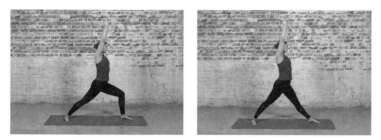

16. WARRIOR 1 IN MOTION: Stand with legs open wide. Turn right foot to point to right side, left foot turns in slightly to right. Then turn body to face the right squarely and raise arms alongside head, palms facing in. Exhaling bend front leg, inhaling extend front leg. Repeat 6-8 times then move directly into Warrior 2 before repeating to left.

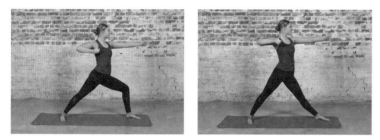

17. WARRIOR 2 IN MOTION: With feet as for Warrior 1, turn hips and shoulders to face forward and pull arms out to sides as if holding a bow and arrow. Thumbs point upwards, fingers curl into palms. Look at extended right arm. Exhaling bend right leg, inhaling extend right leg. Repeat 6-8 times. Then repeat Warrior 1 and 2 to left.

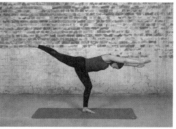
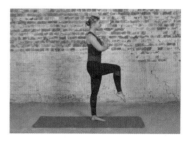

18 WARRIOR 3 IN MOTION: Start standing facing forward with legs open wide. Exhaling, turn to right, bending right knee as reach arms forwards and raise left leg up behind you. Inhaling return to upright, centered position. Repeat to left. Repeat 3-6 times alternating sides.

19. MARCH AND BALANCE: Hold for 3 breaths with right leg raised in marching position, hands in prayer pose. Repeat to left.

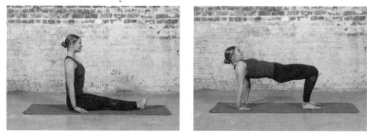

20. DYNAMIC HALF BRIDGE: Sit with legs extended and slightly apart, feet flexed and arms at sides with fingers pointing forwards. Inhaling rock hips forwards with knees and elbows bending, then raise hips up into half bridge, standing into feet, arms extending and looking forwards. Exhaling reverse motion to return to upright sitting position. Repeat 6-8 times.

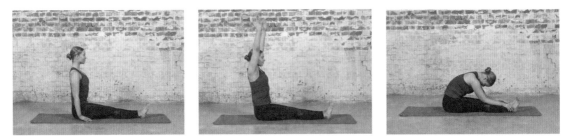

21. FORWARD BEND: Sit upright, arms at sides with legs together and extended, feet flexed. Inhaling, raise arms sideways and up, palms facing in. Exhaling reach forwards from tail bone to fingertips, making your way into full forward bend, taking hold of ankles or feet and lowering head towards knees. Hold for 5 breaths. Then inhaling reverse movements to return to upright sitting position with arms at sides.

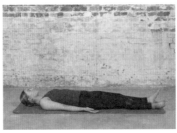

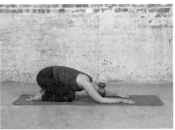

OPTIONAL FOR A MORE INTENSIVE WORKOUT:

Repeat entire strength workout 1 or 2 more times before moving on to rest pose.

22. Rest on back for 10 easy breaths. Then inhale deeply and hum a long "mmmmm" sound, repeating 3 times, to feel the vibration and strength of your voice.

23. From lying on back, stretch out arms and legs, curl onto one side and then move into a child's pose. Relax for a few moments.

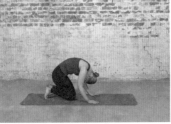

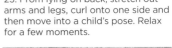

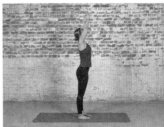

24. TRANSITION TO STANDING: From child's pose shift hips back over feet, curling toes under and then raising hips into forward hang over slightly bent legs. Hold for a few moments then unfold spine to upright, raising arms sideways and up to touch overhead and then bringing arms down to sides.

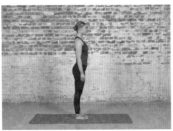

Exercises to Promote Fluidity, Agility and Flexibility and Dopamine's Energising, Inspiring and Motivating Kind of Happiness

'It is not the strongest of the species that survive, nor the most intelligent, but the one most responsive to change.'

CHARLES DARWIN

There are two workout options offered here for developing the physical skills of fluidity, agility and flexibility in different ways. They are designed to boost your ability to respond well to change. One is for boosting creativity and zest for life. This workout loosens you up and brings greater fluidity into your shoulder girdle and hip areas in particular. These areas are associated with your ability to feel more mobile physically that in turn is associated with qualities such as creativity and zest for life. The exercises make use of shaking, twisting, stretching and swinging movements. You will also need to find your centre and strength as you navigate some of the exercises, to be able to keep your balance, which is an important complementary skill to creativity. In addition to loosening up, the creativity workout opens your chest area to enhance inhalation and metaphoric inspiration as well as inviting you to experience heartfelt inspiration.

The next workout is for strengthening your physical reach and perseverance. This workout uses a yoga flow called the sun salutation. It is a classic way to greet the rising sun and can be practised at any time of day. It can help fire up a positive, motivated and perseverant mindset. It invites you to reach through your body's endpoints, which include the crown of your head, your tail bone, hands and feet, as you stretch your body out in various directions. Following the basic version are optional add-ons to vary or intensify your repetitions of the salutation sequence.

Metaphorically, reaching and stretching out your body can take you out of your comfort zone and represent your willingness to dream and reach beyond current horizons towards meaningful aspirations. This workout invites you to also balance your reaching with being grounded through your feet and sometimes your hands, too, for stabilisation. There is also an invitation to coordinate movement with breathing, to mimic the ebb and flow of life and boost perseverance.

Before beginning with these guided workouts, here are a few simple suggestions for focusing specifically on agility to add a spring to your step. Each suggestion below can be performed in the comfort of your own home and in 10 minutes, or longer if you like. You can also use any of these as an add-on to any of the workouts in this book if you want a higher intensity and cardiovascular component. Note that it is important to warm up before moving into high intensity exercise. The first option of running on the spot with star jumps for 5 to 10 minutes can serve as sufficient warm up or, if you are using a skipping rope, you can warm up with 5–10 minutes of easy skipping.

Agility Workout Options for Adding a Spring to Your Step

Time estimate: 10 minutes

Alternate running on the spot (trying to kick your bottom) for a minute or two, with star jumps (or jumping jacks touching or clapping hands overhead when legs jump open and arms down to sides when legs jump together) for a minute or two. Continue this alternation for 5 or 10 minutes depending on your level of fitness and moving at a pace and intensity that is comfortable.

- As you carry this out, find an even rhythm for your breathing. Rhythm can make exertion feel easier and can increase endurance. Maybe you breathe in as you carry out three running movements and breathe out for 3 runs, or 4 or whatever feels comfortable for you. Just find a rhythm that you can keep steady and in time with your running.

- For a higher intensity workout you can use just running on the spot, alternating 30 seconds of high and low intensity. For the high-intensity part, it is helpful to raise your knees up in front of you as you run on the spot as fast as you can. This is instead of kicking your feet up behind you. For the low intensity 30 seconds, return to kicking your feet up behind you or walk around the room for more of a low intensity break. Continue for 5 or 10 minutes depending on your fitness.

- Skipping with a rope will get your heart rate up and your bounce going. Start with 5–10 minutes of low intensity, easy skipping. Then you can increase the intensity by alternating 30 seconds of skipping as fast as you can with 30 seconds of either skipping slowly or walking around the room as you catch your breath. Continue this alternation of high and low intensity movement for 5 or 10 minutes to get your heart rate and fitness going.

Put on some music and dance! As the saying goes: 'dance like nobody's watching'. Any time of the day, dancing for as long as you can, can loosen you up, release tension, let go of pent-up emotions and generate happiness!

Workout for Boosting Creativity and Zest for Life

Time estimate: 20 minutes

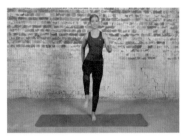

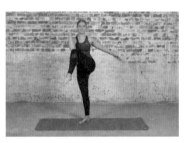

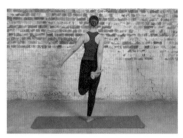

1. March for 20-30 beats on the spot with arms swinging.

2. March 8 times, bringing opposite elbow to knee.

3. March 8 times with legs kicking up behind you to touch opposite hand to foot.

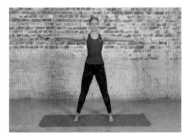

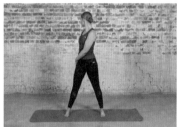

4. Side to side swing with legs a comfortable distance apart and bending knees as swing arms to wrap around hips. Swing from side to side 8 times.

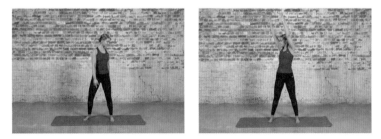

5. Side to side swing with legs a comfortable distance apart. Arms lower with bent knees then legs extend as twist to one side, raising arms up high. Swing from side to side 8 times.

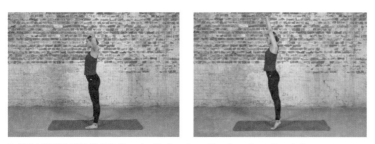

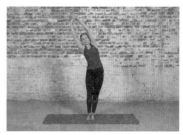

6. STANDING REACHES: Stand with legs together, hands on head, fingers interlaced, palms facing up. Inhaling rise up on toes pressing hands up high and looking up to hands. Exhaling lower to starting position. Repeat 8 times.

7. SIDE BENDS: With fingers interlaced, palms facing up, exhale bending over to one side and inhale returning to upright. Repeat 4 times each side.

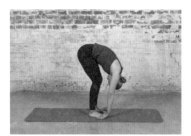

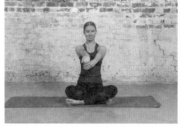

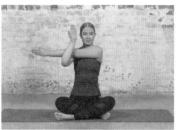

8. FORWARD HANG: With legs hip distance apart and parallel, hang forwards over bent legs for 5 breaths with weight slightly back over heels.

9. HAND-FOREARM STRETCHES: Extend right arm, palm facing forwards. Pull fingers back to stretch front forearm for 2 breaths. Then circle hand a few times. Repeat with other hand.

10. UPPER ARM STRETCH: Right arm across chest, hooking left arm over right for stretch to upper arm. Keep shoulder pressed down. Hold for 3 breaths. Repeat to other side.

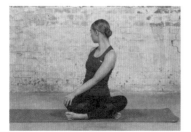

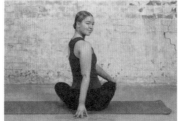

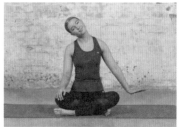

11. SITTING TWIST: Place right hand on left knee and twist to look back over left shoulder. Place left hand on ground behind you. Hold for 2 deep breaths. Repeat to other side.

12. NECK STRETCH: Extend right arm down at angle to the ground with hand flexed. Lower head to left. Hold for 3 breaths. Repeat to other side.

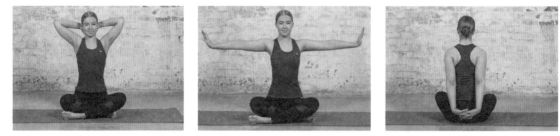

13. ARM AND CHEST STRETCHES: Hook hands behind head, elbows wide and hold for 3 breaths. Reach arms out to sides with hands flexed and hold for 3 breaths. Then hook hands behind hips and extend arms downwards to open chest and hold for 3 breaths.

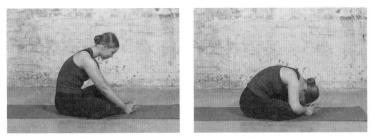

14. Bring feet together in wide butterfly position. Briefly massage legs from hips to toes. Then hold feet and relax forwards over legs, elbows over knees, head relaxing towards feet. Hold for 3 breaths. Then unfold spine to sit upright.

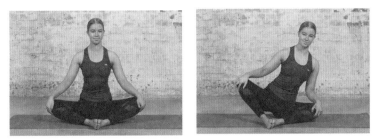

15. BUTTERFLY LEG BOUNCES AND ROCKING: Hold lower legs and bounce knees up and down a few times, then rock from side to side on hips a few times.

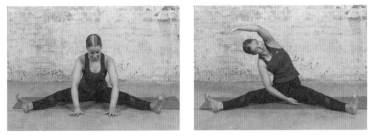

16. SPLIT LEG STRETCHES: Stretch legs out to sides with feet flexed. Reach forwards for stretch to inner thighs and hold for 3-5 breaths. Then return to sit upright and reach over to one side and then the other, holding for 2 breaths each side and repeating side bends 3 times each side.

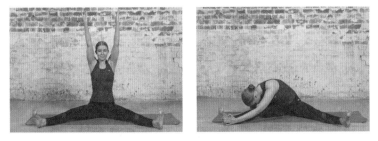

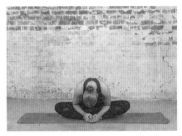

17. FORWARD BEND OVER ONE LEG IN SPLIT POSITION: Inhaling reach arms up and turn to face over right leg. Exhaling reach into forward bend taking hold of right ankle or foot, bringing head towards knee. Hold for 3 breaths. Reverse motion out of position then repeat to other side.

18. BUTTERFLY STRETCH: Bring feet together close in to hips, knees open, elbows over legs, head towards feet. Hold for 5 breaths.

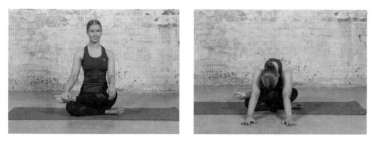

19. CROSS LEG STRETCH: Cross one leg over the other. Bend forwards with arms extended, hands on legs or ground. Hold for 3 breaths. Repeat with other leg on top.

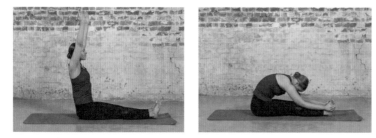

20. FORWARD BEND: Extend both legs in front of you and together, feet flexed. Inhaling reach arms up. Exhaling reach into forward bend holding ankles or feet, head towards knees. Hold for 5 breaths. Reverse motion back to sitting upright.

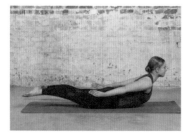
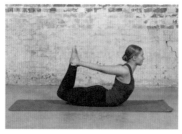

21. BACKWARD ARCH: Lie face down, clasp hands behind hips and reach arms backwards as you raise upper body. Hold for 3-5 breaths.

22. OPTIONAL BOAT POSE: Arch backwards, taking hold of ankles or pointed feet and rock slightly forwards and backwards on belly a few times.

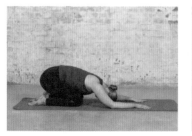
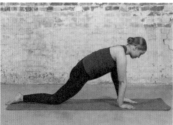

23. CHILD'S POSE INTO HIP STRETCH: Rest in child's pose for 5 breaths. Then move through all fours, bringing right foot forwards between hands. Hold for 3 breaths. Return to child's pose and repeat hip stretch on other side. End in child's pose.

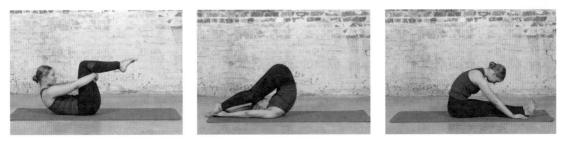

24. ROLLING BALL: Round spine, tuck chin to chest and hook hands under knees. Roll backwards and forwards 8-16 times.

OPTIONAL: Continue for an extra 4 rolls, this time bringing legs and arms overhead when rolling backwards and reaching into forward bend with legs and arms when rolling forwards.

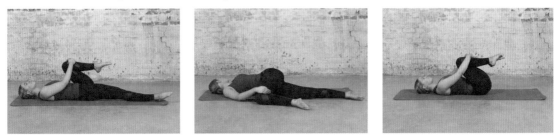

25. SPINAL TWIST LYING DOWN: Lie on back, hug both knees in over belly. Extend left leg on ground and take right knee with left hand. Ease right knee over towards ground on left for spinal twist while extending right arm out to right side, palm on ground. Look to right and hold for 3-5 breaths. Return to lie on back hugging both knees and repeat to left. End with a few rolling balls.

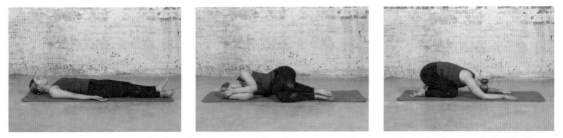

26. Lie comfortably flat on your back, or bend knees with feet flat on ground if you need lower back support. Rest for 8 easy breaths or a few minutes. To transition, wriggle fingers and toes, take a deep breath and stretch, then curl onto your side and move into child's pose for a few moments.

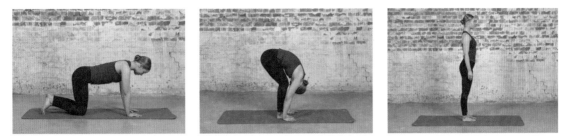

27. TRANSITION TO STANDING: Move onto all fours and shift weight back over feet. Raise hips into relaxed forward bend over slightly bent legs then unfold.

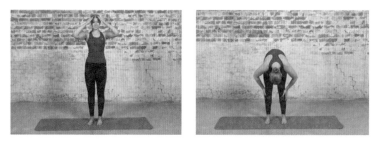

28. ENERGISING BODY SWEEP: Rub hands together then sweep hands over head, down back of body, round feet and up front of body to return to prayer pose. Repeat 3 times.

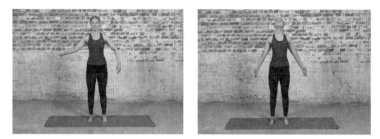

29. Shake out from head to toe, then open arms and hands at sides and raise chest while looking up in the spirit of creative openness. Take 2 deep breaths to close workout.

Workout for strengthening your reach and perseverance №1

Move smoothly from posture to posture in this basic Sun Salutation

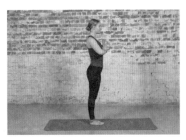

1. Stand in prayer pose.

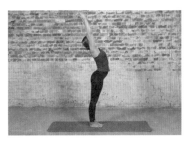

2. Inhaling, reach arms up, palms facing in and bend slightly backwards, looking up.

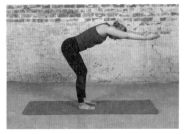

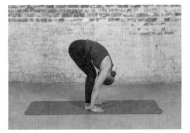

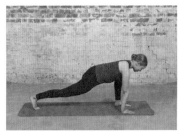

3. Exhaling, reach forwards and down into full forward bend, head towards legs, legs extended or slightly bent.

4. Inhaling, step right leg back.

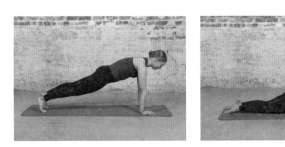

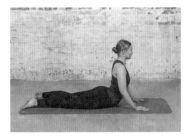

5. Exhaling,step back into plank pose and lower knees, chest and forehead to ground in caterpillar pose. Elbows in at sides.

6. Inhaling, lower hips to ground, arch back and raise head into cobra pose with elbows in at sides.

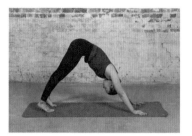

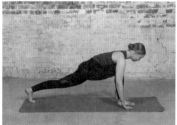

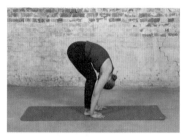

7. Exhaling, raise hips into down-facing dog pose. Heels towards ground.

8. Inhaling,step right foot forwards between hands.

9. Exhaling, step feet together and extend legs as much as possible in full forward bend.

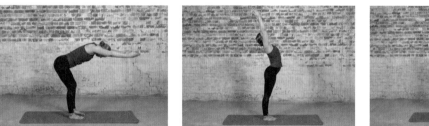

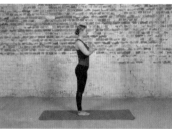

10. Inhaling, reach up through tabletop to upright and lean slightly backwards, looking up to hands.

11. Exhaling, join hands and return to standing prayer pose.

Repeat to the left.

Repeat 3-8 rounds (right and left) or more if you like.

OPTIONAL: Follow this with cooling-down kneeling stretches included later in "stretches and muscle recovery suggestions."

Workout for strengthening your reach and perseverance №2

More strenuous sun salutation option

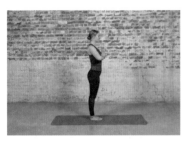

1. Stand in prayer pose.

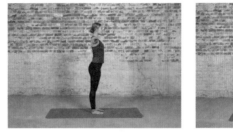

2. Inhaling, reach arms sideways and up to touch overhead, looking up to hands.

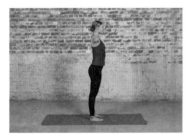

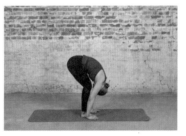

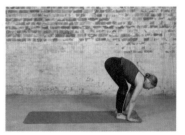

3. Exhaling, reach arms sideways and down into forward bend, hands alongside feet, knees bent if needed.

4. Inhaling, extend spine and reach head forwards with hands alongside feet.

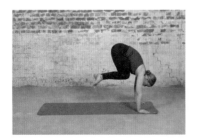

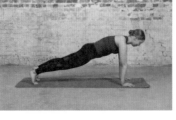

5. Exhaling, jump back to plank position.

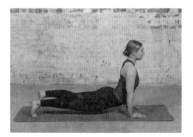

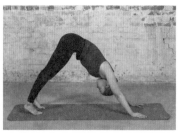

6. Inhaling, lower hips to just above ground and raise upper body into upward-facing dog pose, looking up.

7. Exhaling, raise hips and press back into downward-facing dog pose.

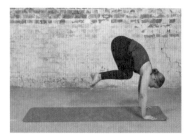

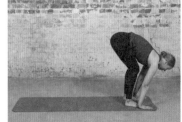

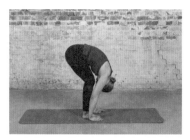

8. Inhaling, jump feet forwards between hands then extend legs as much as possible into forward bend with spine and head reaching forwards.

9. Exhaling, lower spine and head into full forward bend, knees slightly bent if needed.

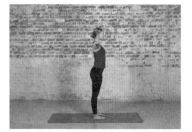

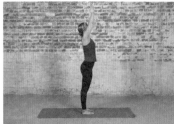

10. Inhaling, unfold spine to upright, reaching arms sideways and up to touch overhead and looking up to hands.

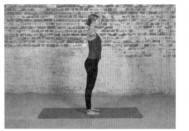

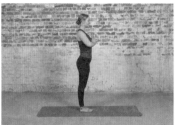

11. Exhaling, lower arms sideways and return to prayer pose.

Repeat 3-6 times. Recommended for use after 3-6 rounds of basic sun salutation for a more intensive workout and recommended to return to basic salutation for 3-6 rounds afterwards too.

Exercises to Promote Warmheartedness and Oxytocin's Connected, Reflected and Heartfelt Kind of Happiness

'When people open their hearts they find the courage to do remarkable things.'

ROBERT M. DRAKE

In this workout you are given many opportunities to bring your chest and 'heart' forwards and build strength in your ability to live a heart-led life. There is also an invitation for you to work at keeping your heart open even when the going gets challenging in some exercises. This can serve as a metaphor for life, inviting you to keep your heart open even when the going gets tough, to inspire heartfelt responding.

You are invited to treat each exercise as an opportunity to breathe into and expand your chest, which houses your heart as well as to strengthen the muscles that can help you feel stronger in your heart-led living. These include your upper body and arm muscles as well as your core.

Heart-opening Workout

Time estimate: 20 minutes

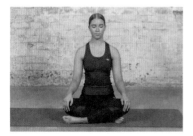

1. Sit comfortably with eyes closed or focused on point on ground and take 3 deep breaths as if breathing through your heart.

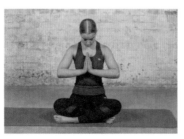

2. Place hands in prayer pose and bow head to hands. Hold for 3 breaths.

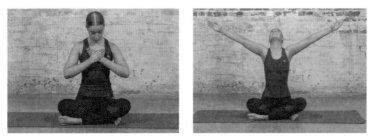

3. CHEST EXPANSION: Place hands on chest. Inhaling open arms wide looking slightly up. Exhaling close hands back to chest looking down. Repeat smoothly 8 times.

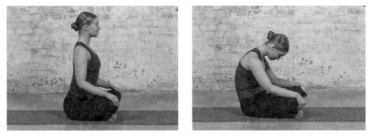

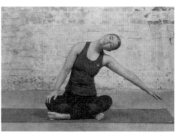

4. SPINE UNDULATION: Inhaling arch spine, bringing chest forwards. Exhaling round spine. Coordinate breath with movement and repeat 8 times.

5. SIDE TO SIDE SWAY TO LOOSEN UP SPINE: Keeping hips centred, sway 8 times from side to side, extending arm out to side.

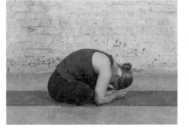

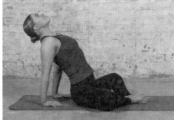

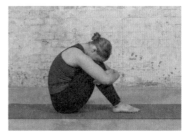

6. SITTING FORWARD-BACKWARD BEND: Feet together in wide butterfly position. Relax forwards over legs, hold feet, elbows over knees. Hold for 3 breaths. Unfold spine to back bend, looking up with hands on ground behind you. Hold for 3 breaths.

7. Hug knees in to chest for 2 breaths.

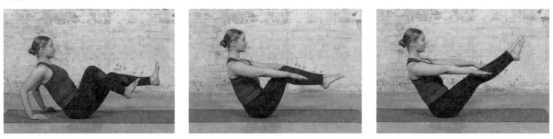

8. SUPPORTIVE CORE STRENGTHENING: Leaning back on arms, cycle legs in front of you 8-16 times.

Optional extra: Bend and stretch legs together, inhaling drawing legs in, exhaling extending legs. Repeat 4-8 times.

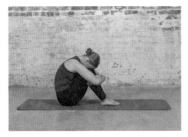

9. Hug knees in to chest for 2 breaths.

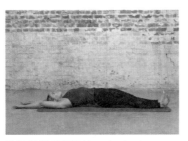

10. BODY STRETCH: Lie on back, raise arms, flex feet, press down in heels and shoulders as raise hips off ground. Hold for 2 breaths then sway hips side to side a few times.

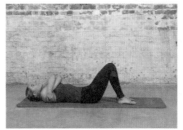

UPPER BACK RELEASE: Lie on back, knees bent. Hug arms across chest, taking hold around shoulders. Rock upper back side to side a few times. Then run hands up back of neck so spine long.

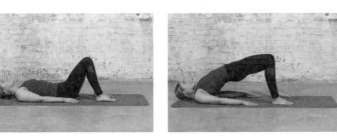

12. HALF BRIDGE: Lie flat on back with knees bent. Inhaling stand into feet and raise hips, peeling spine off ground and bringing chest towards chin. Hold for 3 breaths. Exhaling lower through spine to starting position. Repeat 3 times.

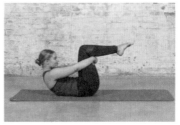

13. ROLLING BALL: Hug knees, round spine, tuck chin in and roll back and forwards a few times for spinal massage.

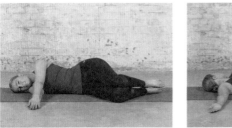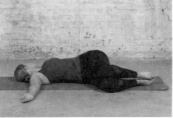

14. GENTLE SPINAL TWIST: Lie on left side, legs bent, arms extended with hands touching. Inhaling open right arm to place on ground on right with palm up, causing twist in upper body. Look to right as hold for 3 breaths. Return to lying on left side. Repeat to other side.

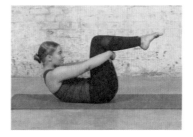

15. ROLLING BALL: Once again hug knees, round spine, tuck chin in and roll back and forwards a few times for spinal massage.

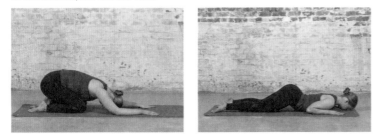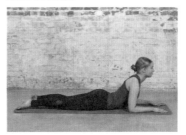

16. CHILD'S POSE INTO LOW COBRA: Rest in child's pose with arms alongside head for 3 breaths. Then inhaling slide forwards and raise upper body into low cobra with forearms on ground. Exhaling move back into child's pose. Repeat 3 times.

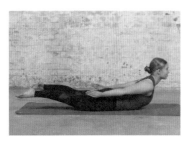

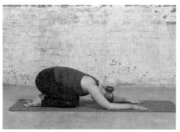

17. BACKWARD ARCH: From lying face down with arms at sides, reach arms and legs backwards and up. Hold for 3 breaths.

18. CHILD'S POSE: Rest for 5 breaths.

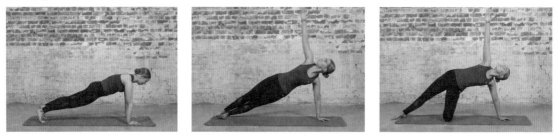

19. PLANK WITH TWIST: Move into plank pose and open one arm up, looking up to top hand if you can otherwise down to ground. Hold for 2-3 breaths. Repeat to other side. If needed, twist from all fours with knee on ground.

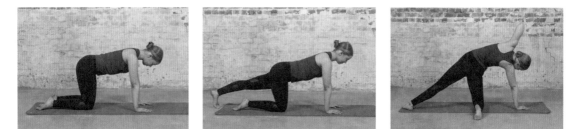

20. EXTENDED TWIST AND STRETCH TO OPEN CHEST: Start on all fours. Extend right leg behind you, toes curled under on ground, and shift left hand slightly out to left side for better balance. Push hips forwards to arch spine, looking down to bottom hand. Then raise right elbow with hand touching right shoulder...

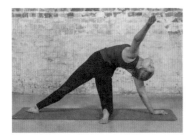

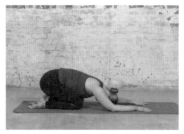

... and from there extend right arm far backwards following spinal arch, as if lying over a barrel. Hold for 2-3 breaths. Reverse movements back to all fours. Repeat to other side.

21. CHILD'S POSE: Rest for 5 breaths.

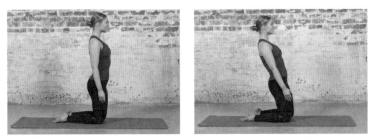

22. KNEELING BACK BENDS: Sit up on knees. Inhaling upright, exhaling lean back aiming for straight line knees to head. Repeat 8 times.

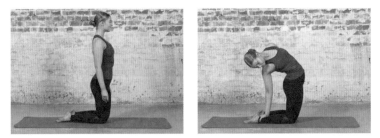

23. REACHING BACK HAND TO HEEL: Inhaling upright, exhaling reach one hand back to touch heel with hips over knees. Repeat 3 times each side.

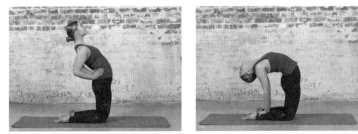
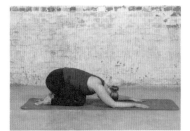

24. KNEELING BACK BEND TO OPEN CHEST: Place hands on hips, drawing elbows and shoulder blades together behind you. Arch backwards and if you can reach both hands back to hold heels. Hold for 2-3 breaths Reverse motion to return to upright.

25. CHILD'S POSE: Rest for 5 breaths.

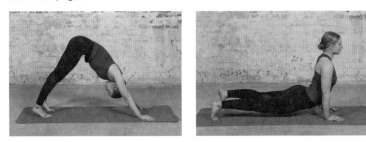
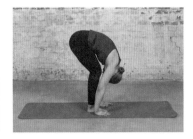

2. Rock between upward- and downward-facing dog, stretch 4-8 times.

27. From downward dog, walk hands back to feet and hang forwards over slightly bent legs for 5 breaths.

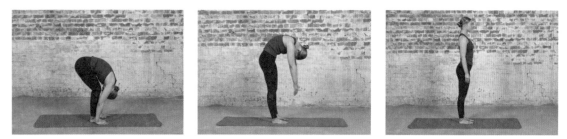

28. Roll up and down spine 3 times, coordinating breath with movement. Inhaling, unfold to upright, extending legs. Exhaling, hang forwards, bending knees slightly.

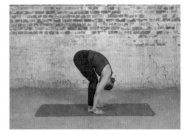 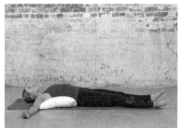 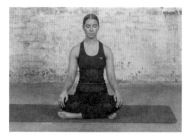

29. OPTIONAL HANDSTAND AGAINST WALL: From standing, kick up to a handstand against a wall. Hold for 3-5 breaths. Or for easier option, face in to wall and walk feet up wall to hold for 1-2 breaths.

30. Hang forwards over slightly bent legs for 3-5 breaths.

31. Rest on back for a few minutes with option of lying over cushion to expand chest area with arms open to sides, palms up.

32. HEART MEDITATION: Sit cross legged, on a cushion if you like. Close eyes or focus on ground and smile from your heart. Take a few minutes to send loving-kindness outwards to others, the world and back to yourself.

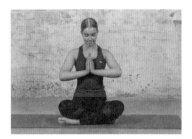

33. Place hands in prayer pose and bow to close heart workout.

Stretches and Muscle Recovery Ideas

In the days following your strength workout or other workouts you might find when you wake that your muscles feel stiff or sore. Following the strength workout in particular, there are a few brief stretches that might be helpful to relieve shoulder and arm stiffness. Or you could repeat the same workout the next day and then on alternate days for a week or so, which can also help your muscles to recover while helping you grow stronger. The creativity workout is also a great one for loosening up tensions that might build up in your body. Also included are a few general suggestions for supporting muscle recovery.

A Few Stretches and Muscle-recovery Suggestions

The arm stretches can be particularly helpful after the strength workout. The kneeling stretches can be particularly helpful after the sun salutation.

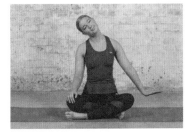

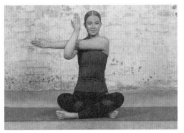

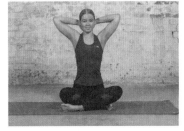

While sitting, extend right arm down at angle to ground with hand flexed. Lean head towards left shoulder for stretch to right side of neck. Hold for 3 breaths.

Extend right arm across chest, hook left arm over right for stretch to right shoulder and upper arm. Hold for 3 breaths. Repeat to other side.

Hook hands behind neck, opening elbows out to sides. Hold for 3 breaths.

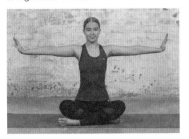

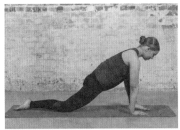

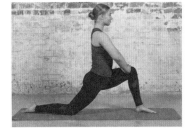

Extend arms out to sides with palms flexed for stretch to arms. Hold for 3 breaths.

Hold lunge stretch for 3-5 breaths each side with hands on ground alongside feet or placed on knee.

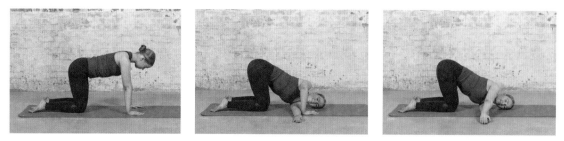

UPPER BACK TWIST: From all fours feed right hand under left and extend along ground, palm up. Place left hand on top of right. Hold for 3-5 breaths. Then reverse motion back to all fours and repeat to other side. End in child's pose with arms at sides for a few easy breaths.

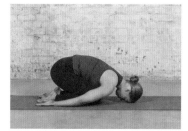

SUPPORTIVE RECOVERY OPTIONS

- Happy posture grounded, fluid movements: The grounded and fluid movements in the section on 'Happy Posture' can help to iron out tension and align your body to avoid further strain from stiffness that can compromise your posture.
- The workout for creativity and zest for life contains stretches and loosening practices for the upper body and the body as a whole.
- Self-holding: The self-hold sequence in the 'Sleep Support' chapter can have a soothing effect.
- Soak in a warm bath, perhaps with bath salts. You can find bath salts for support of muscles recovery at your local health shop or pharmacy.

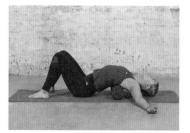 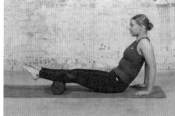

ONE MORE SUPPORTIVE RECOVERY OPTION

- Roll out your muscles: The technical term for this is self-myofacial release. Use a PVC pipe or cylindrical-shaped foam and leverage your own body weight to target the muscles you want to massage. You might be limited to the muscles that you can easily reach, such as in your back. Lie on the cylinder and carefully roll slowly backwards and forwards with your knees bent and your feet on the ground for support.
- You can also roll over the muscles at the backs of your legs by sitting with your extended legs balanced on the roller and shifting your weight slowly forwards and backwards over the roller for a massage to your calf muscles and the backs of your thighs. Even if you roll out just these areas, it can provide welcome relief as a massage might do.

You can try self-myofacial release for 5 minutes or so after exercise as part of winding down, or you can include it for 5-10 minutes on a break day from exercising.

Sourcing a roller: you should be able to source the foam option from a sports store, a physiotherapy practice or a Pilates studio. The PVC pipe you can buy from the hardware store and ask them to cut to a size of about 18 inches or 46 centimetres in length, and 4.5 inches or 11.5 centimetres in diameter. Even though a foam roller can be softer on the body, as you get used to the hardness of a PVC pipe it can get into sore spots really effectively.

SOURCES AND NOTES

The Bio-chemistry and Physical Skills of Happiness

BBC documentary: *The Ghost in Your Genes* available as free online documentary through https://ihavenotv.com/the-ghost-in-your-genes

Benson, H. (1975, updated 2001). *The Relaxation Response*. HarperCollins: USA

Fry, A.C., Schilling, B.K., Fleck, S.J. and Kraemer, W.J. (January 2011). 'Relationships between competitive wrestling success and neuroendocrine responses', *Journal of Strength and Conditioning Research,* 25(1): 40–45

Pert, C. (1999). *Molecules of Emotion: The Science behind Mind-Body Medicine*. Touchstone: New York

Yehuda, R. et al. (1998). 'Phenomenology and Psychobiology of the Intergenerational Response to Trauma' in *Yael Danieli, Intergenerational Handbook of Multigenerational Legacies of Trauma*. Plenum: New York

Grounding

Bujatti, M. and Biederer, P. (September 1976). 'Serotonin, noradrenaline, dopamine metabolites in transcendental meditation-technique', *Journal of Neural Transmission,* 39(3): 257-267

Chevalier, G., Sinatra, S.T., Oschman, J.L., Sokal, K. and Sokal, P. (published online 12 January 2012). 'Earthing: Health Implications of Reconnecting the Human Body to the Earth's Surface Electrons' in Journal of Environmental and Public Health, 29154

Creswell, J.D., Taren, A.A., Lindsay, E.K., Greco, C.M., Gianaros, P.J., Fairgrieve, A., Marsland, A.L., Brown, K.W., Way, B.M., Rosen, R.K. and Ferris, J.L. (1 July 2016) . 'Alterations in Resting-State Functional Connectivity Link Mindfulness Meditation With Reduced Interleukin-6: A Randomized Controlled Trial' in *Biological Psychiatry,* 80(1): 53-61

Levine, P. A. (2010). *In An Unspoken Voice: How the Body Releases Trauma and Restores Goodness.* North Atlantic Books: California

Roth, T., Mayleben, D., Feldman, N., Lankford, A., Timothy, G. and Nofzinger, E. (2018). 'A novel forehead temperature-regulating device for insomnia: A randomized clinical trial' in Sleep, 41.10.1093/sleep/zsy045

Toshiyo T., Kumi H., Masao T. and Norito K. (2007). 'The Immediate Effects of 10-minute Relaxation Training on Salivary Immunoglobulin A (s-Ig-A) and Mood State for Japanese Female Medical Co-Workers' in *Acta Medica Okayama,* 61(3): 139-145
For more detail about the World Health Organization's classification of burnout, refer to https://www.who.int/mental_health/evidence/burn-out/en/

Oschman, J.L., Chevalier, G. Brown, R. (March 2015). 'The effects of grounding (earthing) on inflammation, the immune response, wound healing, and prevention and treatment of chronic inflammatory and autoimmune diseases' in *Journal of Inflammation Research* 8(default): 83–96.

Strength

Hung, I.W. Labroo, A.A. (2010). 'From Firm Muscles to Firm Willpower: Understanding the Role of Embodied cognition in Self-Regulation' in *Journal of Consumer Research,* 37(6): 1046-1064

Levine, P.A. (2010). *In An Unspoken Voice: How the Body Releases Trauma and Restores Goodness.* North Atlantic Books: California

For a brief overview of some research linking exercise and testosterone in men and women, refer to online article written by Tim Jewell, medically reviewed by Daniel Bubnis, MS, NASM-CPT, NASE Level II-CSS, specialty in fitness, on 26 September 2019 titled: Does Working Out Increase Testosterone Levels? https://www.healthline.com/health/does-working-out-increase-testosterone

Fluidity, Agility, Flexibility

Beaty, RE., Kenett YN., Christensen A.P., Rosenberg, M.D., Benedek, M., Chen, Q., Fink A., Qiu J., Kwapil T.R., Kane M.J. and Silva P.J. (2018 January). 'Robust prediction of individual creative ability from brain functional connectivity' in Proceedings of the National Academy of Sciences, 115(5):1087–1092.

Goldin-Meadow, Susan, TEDx UChicago presentation on Youtube: What Our Hands Can Tell Us About Our Minds

Miles, Lynden K., Nind, Louise K. Macrae, Neil. (8 January 2010). 'Moving Through Time: Thinking of the past or future causes us to sway backward or forward' in Association for Psychological Science, January 8, 2010.

Opezzo, M. and Schwartz, D. (April 2014). 'Give Your Ideas Some Legs: The Positive Effect of Walking on Creative Thinking' in *Journal of Experimental Psychology: Learning, Memory and Cognition,* 40(4).

Shafir, T. (2015). 'Body-based strategies for emotion regulation' in M.L. Bryant (Ed.), *Handbook on Emotion Regulation: Processes, Cognitive Effects and Social Consequences* (pp 231-249). Nova Science Publishers, Inc.

Shafir, T. and Tsachor, R. (January 2016). 'Emotion Regulation through Movement: Unique Sets of Movement Characteristics are Associated with and Enhance Basic Emotions' in *Frontiers in Psychology,* 6(188).

Slepian, M.L. and Ambady, N. (February 2012). 'Fluid Movement and Creativity' in *Journal of Experimental Psychology: General,* 141(4).

Warmheartedness

Kok, B.E. and Fredrickson, B.L. (2010). 'Upward spirals of the heart: autonomic flexibility, as indexed by vagal tone, reciprocally and prospectively predicts positive emotions and social connectedness' in *Biological Psychology*, 85, 432–436, ISBN 1873–62460

To find out more about The HeartMath Institute, refer to heartmath.org

Neff, K. To find out more about mindful self-compassion and the work of Dr Kristin Neff refer to https://self-compassion.org/

Shaltout, H.A., Tooze, J.A., Rosenberger, E. Kemper, K.J. (May 2012). 'Time, Touch, and Compassion: Effects on Autonomic Nervous System and Well-Being' in *Explore, The Journal of Science and Healing,* 8(3):177–84.

Bouncing Back from Stress and Maintaining Happiness

Boser, A. (2016). *Undulation: Relieve stiffness and feel younger*, second edition. Vital Self, Incorporated

Dana, Deb. (2018). *The Polyvagal Theory in Therapy: Engaging the Rhythm of Regulation.* New York: W. W. Norton & Company

Kalyani, B.G., Venkatasubramanian, G., Arasappa, R. Rao, N.P., Kalmady, S.V., Behere, R.V., Rao, H., Vasudev M.K., Gangadhar, B.N. (2011). 'Neurohemodynamic correlates of "OM" chanting. A pilot functional magnetic resonance imaging study' in *International Journal of Yoga,* 4(1): 3–6

Kennedy, J. (2012). 'Neurocardiac and Neuro-biofeedback Measurement of Financial Executive Performance as Associated with HRV Metrics' in *Neuroleadership Journal,* 4: 81-87

As an introduction to the 'tend and befriend' stress response: Taylor, S., Klein, L., Lewis, B., Gruenwald, T., Gurung, R. and Updegraff, J. (2000) 'Biobehavioral Responses to Stress in Females: TendandBefriend, Not FightorFlight' in *Psychological Review*, 107(3): 411-429

Kok, B.E. Coffey, K.A., Cohn, M.A., Catalino, L.I., Vacharkulksemsuk, T.S., Algoe, B., Brantley, M. Fredrickson, B.L. (May 2013) 'How Positive Emotions Build Physical Health: Perceived Positive Social Connections Account for the Upward Spiral Between Positive Emotions and Vagal Tone' in *Psychological Science,* 24(7)

Porges, S.W. (1995). 'Orienting in a defensive world: Mammalian modifications of our evolutionary heritage: A Polyvagal Theory' in *Psychophysiology,* 32: 301-318

Porges, Stephen W. (2018). 'Connectedness as a Biological Imperative: Understanding trauma through the lens of Polyvagal Theory', interview for the Healing Trauma Summit. Louisville, CO: Sounds True

Stellar, J.E., Cohen, A., Oveis, C. and Keltner, D. (2015). 'Affective and physiological responses to the suffering of others: compassion and vagal activity' in *Journal of Personality and Social Psychology*, 108(4)

About the Author

International best-selling author and psychologist Noa Belling uses her many years' experience of intellectual and physical discipline to guide others in enhancing vitality and life fulfilment. Noa holds a Masters degree in somatic (body-mind) psychology through Naropa University. Her background includes many years of running a private psychotherapy practice and presenting talks, workshops and executive coaching in the business world. She has also taught applied somatic psychology skills for many years as part of psychology training and continuing education programs.

Noa's first career as a professional ballet dancer and then a yoga teacher also influence her approach to wellbeing. Her personal journey in physical intelligence started as a ballet dancer, a period that spanned over 20 years of her early life and included a few years as a professional dancer. Through dance, she regularly experienced backstage nerves dissolving into physical control, poise and presence in the moment of stepping out onstage. Dance regularly filled her with joy while strengthening, stretching and grounding her body in ways that supported her resilience and topped up her happiness through life's ups downs. In her twenties she discovered yoga and meditation, both of which added a mindful grounding and centring element to her dancer physical intelligence. Noa went on to pursue academic studies in psychology and dance or movement as therapy, leading to her masters degree. This experience enhanced her ability to blend Western and Eastern approaches to psychology and personal mastery.

Noa feels passionately about sharing and teaching skills that draw on the body, especially as it has played such a core and empowering role in her life. Her work strives to elevate the value of body awareness in society, to be better recognised as the powerful change agent that it can be. This involves expanding body awareness beyond the realms of physical exercise and nutrition, and to include all the rich ways that we can draw on physical intelligence to support us psychologically – in this case supporting our pursuit of happiness.

Noa's journey as a published author began in 2001 with her yoga books, including the international bestseller *The Yoga Handbook* and other titles. More recently Noa wrote *The Mindful Body* (Rockpool publishes, 2018) as a valuable resource for building emotional strength and managing stress with body mindfulness. *The Happiness Workout* is a continuation of this commitment to sharing practical, inspiring body-based skills.

Other products by Noa Belling

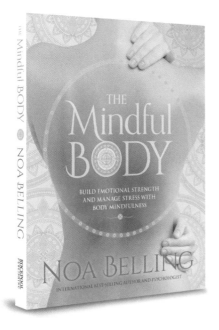

THE MINDFUL BODY
Build Emotional Strength and Manage Stress with Body Mindfulness
ISBN: 978-1-925682-18-2

How does your mind live in your body? How can body awareness change your life experience?
Successful author and practising psychotherapist Noa Belling offers a practical, personal way to use your body as a direct path to mindfulness and mindful living. By waking up to how we hold life experiences in our bodies, we have the power and choice to improve physical, mental and emotional health, promote vitality, build emotional resilience and generally improve quality of life.

The practises of this book go beyond traditional mindfulness to target specific challenges such as stress, anxiety, depression, confidence, zest for life, decision-making and more. Supported with psychological and neuroscientific studies, this book provides you with many opportunities to practise body mindfulness to experience your physical being as an empowering and intelligent resource.

Acknowledgements

Firstly I would like to thank Rockpool Publishing for giving life to this book. I feel so grateful to be part of the Rockpool family, which represents so many inspiring voices. I extend a special thank you to editor Katie Day for her big part in shaping and refining The Happiness Workout and my previous book, The Mindful Body, too. I truly appreciate your input and the clear value that you add. Thank you to Sarah Dennett for beautifully and patiently demonstrating all of the workout postures, to Katie Rose for supervising Sarah on the photoshoot, to Paul Robbins of Monde Photo for the excellent photography, and to the Rockpool team for coordinating and providing a venue for the shoot. Thank you also to Sara Lindberg for the magnificent book design and the focus and care showed throughout the process of pulling it all together.

I wish to thank all my clients who I have learned so much from and who make my work so fulfilling. To those whose stories are included in this book, sincere thank you for your willingness to share. Thank you to all my teachers along the way, including those I have had the privilege of studying with in person and those whose material in the form of books and online courses has inspired and enriched me personally and professionally.

On a personal note I am so grateful to my family for many things that include being patient with me when I needed to write for hours, sometimes on weekends and whenever I had the chance. I would like to thank my husband, Stephen, for his unwavering love, support and belief in me. I am also so grateful for our two daughters, Emmah and Miela, who regularly top up our happiness reserves, filling our hearts with joy and inspiring us to rise above challenges in parenting and in life.

Finally I would like to thank you, the reader, for investing your time and interest in reading this book. I hope that it inspires and empowers your happiness and yields many rewards.

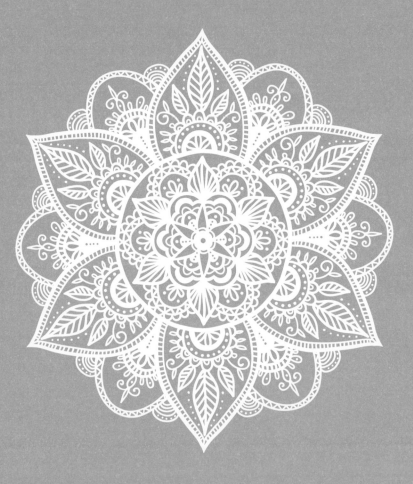